Health Essentials

Vitamin Guide

Hasnain Walji is a writer and freelance journalist specializing in health, nutrition and complementary therapies with a special interest in dietary supplements. A contributor to several journals on environmental and Third World consumer issues, he was the founder and editor of *The Vitamin Connection* – an international journal, published in the UK, Canada and Australia, focusing on the link between health and diet. He also launched *Healthy Eating*, a consumer magazine focusing on the concept of a well-balanced diet, and has written the script for a six part television series, *The World of Vitamins*, that covers nutrition and micronutrient therapy.

The Health Essentials Series

There is a growing number of people who find themselves attracted to holistic or alternative therapies and natural approaches to maintaining optimum health and vitality. The *Health Essentials* series is designed to help the newcomer by presenting high quality introductions to all the main complementary health subjects. Each book presents all the essential information on each therapy, explaining what it is, how it works and what it can do for the reader. Advice is also given, where possible, on how to begin using the therapy at home, together with comprehensive lists of courses and classes available worldwide.

The *Health Essentials* titles are all written by practising experts in their fields. Exceptionally clear and concise, each text is supported by attractive illustrations.

Series Medical Consultant
Dr John Cosh MD, FRCP

In the same series

Acupuncture by Peter Mole
Alexander Technique by Richard Brennan
Aromatherapy by Christine Wildwood
Flower Remedies by Christine Wildwood
Massage by Stewart Mitchell
Reflexology by Inge Dougans with Suzanne Ellis
Shiatsu by Elaine Liechti
Skin and Body Care by Sidra Shaukat
Spiritual Healing by Jack Angelo

Health Essentials

VITAMIN GUIDE

Essential Nutrients
for Healthy Living

HASNAIN WALJI

E L E M E N T

Shaftesbury, Dorset ● Rockport, Massachusetts

Brisbane, Queensland

© Hasnain Walji 1992

Published in Great Britain in 1992 by
Element Books Limited
Longmead, Shaftesbury, Dorset

Published in the USA in 1992 by
Element, Inc
42 Broadway, Rockport, MA 01966

Published in Australia in 1992 by
Element Books Limited for
Jacaranda Wiley Limited
33 Park Road, Milton, Brisbane, 4064

Cover illustration from an Eric Gill woodcut
Cover design by Max Fairbrother
Typeset by The Electronic Book Factory Ltd, Fife, Scotland
Printed and bound in Great Britain by
Dotesios Ltd, Trowbridge, Wiltshire

British Library Cataloguing in Publication
data available

Library of Congress Cataloging in Publication
data available

ISBN 1–85230–375–1

Note from the Publisher
Any information given in any book in the *Health Essentials* series is not intended to be taken as a replacement for medical advice. Any person with a condition requiring medical attention should consult a qualified medical practitioner or suitable therapist.

Contents

Acknowledgements

I would like to express my gratitude to Angela Dowden for her painstaking review of the manuscript and for offering many pertinent suggestions; also to Dr Ahmed Hassam for his constant encouragement and support, and to Christina Ryder without whose contribution, in research and sub-editing, it would have been impossible to write this book.

Last but not least, I wish to thank my wife Latifa whose gentle care and concern enabled me to complete this book.

Introduction

You are what you eat
Anon

FEW PEOPLE WOULD ARGUE with that old adage. We truly *are* what we eat, and these days that includes pesticides on our crops, chemicals added to our food, and poisons in our water.

Concern that twentieth-century environmental factors and a Western lifestyle result in a deficiency of vital nutrients is well founded in the light of maladies that are on the increase; and scientific research abounds with studies confirming that the human body functions best when supplemented with the right nutrients in the correct proportions.

Maintaining good health requires that we adopt a far more positive approach to combat the effect of the destructive barrage which afflicts our bodies day after day, year after year. A close watch on our nutrition intake will reap positive benefits, while to disregard nutritional advice may court disaster. Popular debate, however, is not so clear as to whether we can rely on a well balanced diet alone, or whether we should take nutritional supplements as well.

This book is an attempt to help you disperse the mists of confusion. More importantly, it is concerned with defining the symptoms of health rather than those of disease.

PART ONE
VITAMINS, MINERALS AND SUPPLEMENTS

1

Why We All Need Vitamins and Minerals

Your food is your medicine
Hippocrates (460–370 BC)

'HEALTHY PEOPLE don't really need vitamin supplements.'
'Only pregnant women, nursing mothers and people with specific ailments require supplements.'

'You get all the vitamins and minerals you need from a well balanced diet.'

Ask your GP about vitamin or mineral supplementation and almost invariably the above answers will gush forth with great conviction. But let's take a closer look at two of the key phrases in these statements to see whether we really do need food supplements.

'HEALTHY PEOPLE'

Just what do we mean by the word 'healthy'? All too often we use the word merely to describe the absence of disease: you haven't got cancer or heart disease, and you never miss a day at work, so you must be healthy. But perhaps you are constantly tired, feel run down, catch one cold after another, are listless and unable to do anything after work except flop in front of the TV – despite those good intentions to play squash or go for a long brisk walk. If you are not full of energy, vitality and enthusiasm, can you really consider yourself to be healthy? Then again to consider oneself healthy despite suffering from obesity, insomnia, heartburn,

3

fatigue, low sex drive or premenstrual tension is to misunderstand the term 'health'. Real health is freedom from such frequent minor complaints. Health is far more than the absence of disease – it is a positive state of well-being.

How Healthy Are You?

Health means:

- Being able to work all day and still have the energy left to make the most of an evening out.
- Coping with pressures and stress.
- Having an alert and active mind.
- Resisting infections. This shows that your immune system is operating at par. A number of infections are related to deficiencies of various vitamins.
- Looking healthy. Health and beauty go hand in hand: the condition of one's skin and hair reflect the quality of one's diet.

To maintain health is a permanent challenge, and correct nutrition is a key player in meeting this challenge.

'A WELL-BALANCED DIET'

The generally accepted view is that we can get all the vitamins and minerals we need if we eat a well-balanced diet. But what is a well-balanced diet, and is it actually easy and practical to follow? How many times do you skip breakfast as you rush to work? How often do you grab a burger as you dash back to the office after shopping during your lunch-hour? As you plod home in the evening, a take-away seems so tempting because you are too tired to cook a meal. So when do you have a well-balanced diet? In this fast and frantic rat-race, we need to safeguard our nutritional well-being more than ever before.

By definition a well-balanced diet is one which provides us with the correct proportions of all the nutrients needed by the body. All foods contain varying amounts of nutrients. Proteins, carbohydrates and fats are generously provided in the modern Western diet. These are called macronutrients and form the bulk of the food we eat.

Vitamins and minerals should also be present in the foods we eat. These are known as micronutrients and, as their name implies, are only needed in the body in tiny quantities. These micronutrients are vital ingredients in a healthy diet, and the body cannot function optimally if they are missing. In fact, it has been proven beyond any doubt that if a particular vitamin or mineral is not getting into the system, sooner or later illness will develop.

It would be tempting to think that, as the body only requires vitamins and minerals in small amounts, it is easy enough to fulfil our nutritional requirements, but this is not true. Micronutrients are highly delicate and easily destroyed by a host of factors such as storage, preservation and cooking methods. Also, some vitamins rely on other nutrients if the body is to absorb them and so reap their full nutritional benefit.

Macronutrients, on the other hand, are far less destructible, and therefore our diets tend not to fall short on these 'bulk' foods – proteins, fats and carbohydrates. However, it is becoming increasingly apparent that in the West we are often deficient in micronutrients, and that this is having an adverse effect on our health. Several surveys illustrate that the British public may be falling short on even the most basic nutritional requirements; for further information on this point, turn to page 7.

What Do Vitamins and Minerals Do?

Micronutrients do not contain calories nor provide energy – that is done by the macronutrients. However, this energy cannot be released unless the micronutrients are present. This is because vitamins and minerals form part of the enzymes, the organic catalysts which allow biological processes to take place. This is why vitamins are sometimes called co-enzymes. Human life without enzymes and vitamins would be impossible as they are responsible for converting our food to energy, stimulating the metabolic process and accelerating biological functions.

Vitamins are also involved in growth, in detoxifying the body, in enabling reproduction to take place, and in promoting longevity. Each vitamin plays one or several roles in various aspects of the body's health.

Minerals (such as potassium, magnesium, zinc, selenium and so on) are all around us in the natural world, in rocks and the sea, and they are important for healthy bones and teeth. Like vitamins, minerals cannot be manufactured by the body and must therefore be included in the diet.

Recommended Daily Allowances

Basically we all need the same vitamins and minerals for good health and well-being. However, because individual requirements vary with age, sex, lifestyle, occupation, and exposure to stress and pollution, there can be no general formula to determine our individual needs. There are tables which give average nutrient requirements but these are inadequate because of the manner in which they have been calculated, and because, despite periodic revision, they do not include all known nutrients and are therefore incomplete. These tables are called Recommended Daily Allowances (RDA).

RDA levels are calculated by observing statistically the average food intake of healthy persons and calculating their vitamin and mineral content. For good measure a safety margin is added. Standards in the form of Recommended Intakes for Nutrients (DHSS 1969) and Recommended Daily Allowances (DHSS 1979) have existed in the United Kingdom for over thirty years. However, most of us do not understand how these have been derived, how they are intended to be used, or the degree of accuracy that ought to be attributed to them. In particular the RDAs have commonly (though incorrectly) been used to assess the inadequacy of an individual's diet.

Therefore, in order to overcome the 'abuses' of the figures and to update them in the light of recent information and research, the Department of Health asked the Committee on Medical Aspects of Food Policy (COMA) to set up a panel of experts to look into the matter. As a result a new set of updated figures (collectively known as Dietary Reference Values) has been established, so instead of simple RDA figures we now have four different sets of figures for each nutrient. These are:

- Estimated Average Requirement.
- Recommended Nutrient Intake.
- Lowest Nutrient Intake.
- Safe Intake.

The publication of these new dietary guidelines reflects the fact that at long last the health authorities accept that our individual requirements of specific nutrients differ.

Surveys on Correct Vitamin and Mineral Levels

Recent surveys indicate that the British public may not be attaining the correct vitamin and mineral levels despite believing that we are eating a balanced diet.

In one survey the dietary vitamin and mineral intake was measured in people being given personal advice on good eating habits from a nutritionist. In view of the fact that these people had received expert attention, one would have thought their vitamin and mineral intake would be adequate. Yet, for every nutrient measured, there was a percentage of people who failed to meet the Recommended Daily Allowance. Deficiencies were generally worse in women as they tended to eat less.

Even hospital diets have been found to be lacking in vitamins and minerals. Elderly patients are particularly vulnerable as they are poor eaters. An investigation into the vitamin B intake of the elderly revealed that they selected meals which, even if completely consumed, provided only half of the current recommendation for vitamin B6, and a third of the recommendation for folic acid. Low levels were also recorded for the other B vitamins.

The most overwhelming support for supplementation has come from dietary analysis, in which time and again the diets of individuals have been shown to be lacking in vitamins and minerals. For example, the Dietary and Nutritional Survey of British Adults (HMSO 1990) illustrates that although the average intake of vitamins and minerals in the UK population is usually adequate, significant numbers of subgroups of the population have marginal intakes. According to this report, 2.5 per cent of British women between the ages of twenty-five and thirty-four are only getting 11.8mg or less of vitamin C per day. The recommended figure for this group is 40mg. This means that some 700,000 women are at virtually clinically deficient levels of vitamin C intake!

Similar statistics exist for many other nutrients. As already pointed out, in many cases it is women rather than men who fall short of vitamins and minerals, but there are instances where 2.5 per cent of the entire population (both men and women) fall below the Recommended Daily Allowance. This may not appear significant, but what it means in real terms is that 1.4 million British people are deficient in one or more nutrients.

Finding the Nutrients

No doubt you have heard it said before that the body is like a machine. In some way this is an accurate simile, for just as a car requires petrol, oil, water and regular servicing for it to run smoothly, so our bodies need food and water if they are to operate efficiently. Consider also that it is not enough to put *any* grade of fuel in your car's tank: if you fill it with two-star petrol when it requires four-star, the effect will be noticeable. In the same way, the human body needs the right food and drink for it to function well.

The most important question of all is whether we really are getting all the nutrients we need from our food. There are reasons for believing that we may not be getting all the nourishment we need, even if we are making the right food choices.

We need to realize that vitamins cannot be manufactured by the body and must therefore come from our diet. Indeed nature intended that all the nutrients essential for health be obtained from the food we eat, but what nature proposed, man, with his greed for high productivity and obsession for efficiency, has deposed. Vitamins are delicate, unstable entities that can easily be destroyed during the many processing methods used in modern food production. On its way from the farm to the factory to the supermarket, food is further depleted of essential vitamins and minerals; and what little is left is then lost during its journey from the freezer to the microwave to the table.

Today's science of food manufacture may have produced cheap, plentiful food, but it has also adversely affected the quality of that food. Modern farming techniques employ artificial fertilizers, pesticides and crop sprays, so that the food which is harvested is not only grown in chemicals but is also covered in them. And the soil in which our food is grown is exhausted ('crop rotation is not economical when all the land can be used to produce food'), and consequently deficient in its former natural nutrients.

After harvesting, the produce is treated to give it an extended life to survive the transport, storage and shelf times required by today's food manufacturers. We then store the food at home and often use cooking methods which leach out any vitamin or mineral content which may have remained. The end result is produce which looks and possibly tastes the same as it did fifty years ago (although many would argue this point), but which has little, if any, nutritional value. You may be dutifully eating up your greens, but are they providing you with any goodness?

The Link Between Vitamins and Today's Modern Diseases

It is now accepted that the main cause of many of today's modern diseases is not eating a diet that provides us with the necessary nutrients. And there is little doubt that diet is linked to the increase in the incidence of the major degenerative diseases such as heart disease, osteoporosis, cancer, and many others.

A recent World Health Organization report advocates a daily intake of 400g (approximately 1lb) of fruit and vegetables to include pulses, seeds, and nuts, to keep us healthy. The report also underlines the fact that since the typical Western diet is lacking in sufficient quantities of essential nutrients, we may be overfed but still remain undernourished.

So how do vitamins and other nutrients affect positive health? If you simply consider for a moment that vitamin C is linked to warding off the common cold, the vitamin B-complex to a healthy nervous system, and garlic to lowering blood cholesterol, the connection between diet and true health begins to emerge.

Vitamins and minerals do not just offer day-to-day benefits. There is growing evidence to suggest that some of these micronutrients can also help to prevent the long-term illnesses such as cancer. Vitamins C, E, and beta carotene are now considered to be the main players in this connection.

There is growing speculation that the people least likely to develop cancer are those with the highest blood concentrations of beta carotene, vitamin C and vitamin E, all of which are antioxidants. An antioxidant is a substance that can protect foods from going rancid, and which prevents oxygen from combining with other substances and thus damaging cells. This has led to the widespread belief among researchers that antioxidants may help ward off cancer.

Many of the B vitamins play a vital role in releasing energy from the cells, and stress depletes them much more quickly from the body. The first part of the body to be affected by a mild vitamin B deficiency is the nervous system resulting in anxiety, irritability and depression.

Minerals are close companions for vitamins, in that they act as cofactors and catalysts inside our human cells and have far-reaching effects on our health. Until a few years ago calcium, phosphorus, iron and iodine were recognized as being essential minerals for human health, but as research continues, many more, such as zinc, chromium, magnesium, potassium, manganese and selenium, have joined the ranks.

Ignorance may be bliss, but knowledge of how minerals can make the difference between sickness and health is of great importance, and new findings are bringing to light many ailments caused by mineral deficiencies. Take premenstrual tension (PMT) as an example. Many women find that simply by altering their diet so that it contains more magnesium and zinc, their symptoms can be lessened. Indeed the *Women's Nutritional Advisory Service* has advised many severe PMT sufferers to take the dietary-change-plus-supplementation route, with considerable success. Similar results have been achieved with selenium for rheumatoid arthritis, zinc for skin problems, and calcium for osteoporosis, to name but a few.

As research continues to enhance our understanding of the functions of micronutrients, the importance of maintaining optimum levels of nutrient intake becomes increasingly evident. For example, even marginal deficiencies of vitamins A, C, E, and B6 have been shown to increase susceptibility to a number of viral and bacterial infections. Research indicates that these vitamins help to maintain our immune systems, and that deficiency can impair the body's ability to resist disease.

Dr Willard A. Krehl, of Jefferson Medical College, and Editor-in-Chief of the American *Journal of Clinical Nutrition,* offers the following view:

> My own bias on the value of nutrient supplementation has developed over the years through my experience in clinical practice. I continually see that in spite of the fact that our clients are generally in the executive category and can therefore purchase an excellent diet, most of them do not eat properly. For whatever reasons, most of them skip breakfast or eat the wrong things for breakfast; they have a fast-food lunch high in fat and often low in micronutrients; they consume a good deal of sugar, sweets and alcoholic beverages. In short, my search for the individuals who consistently eat a well balanced, varied and nutritionally adequate diet has merely impressed me with the fact that millions of people do not . . . I strongly

favour multivitamin supplementation and recommend it to my patients because I believe it is a simple, economical, and highly practical way to insure they receive 100 per cent of the RDA for essential micronutrients, and because I believe these intakes are important to health and well-being.

He concludes that

. . . the high incidence of below RDA micronutrient intakes, resulting from multiple factors including poor food choices, decreased caloric intakes and personal/ environmental/lifestyle factors, presents a situation where multivitamin supplementation is both a rational and beneficial choice. Supplementation provides a practical and economic means of insuring adequate nutrient intakes and is of particular importance to risk groups such as dieters, the elderly, heavy drinkers, chronic drug users and others whose diets are insufficient or whose ability to utilize food is impaired . . . I see absolutely no reason to tolerate nutrient inadequacies when such a simple and sensible alternative as a multivitamin exists.

It is important to remember that supplements cannot replace a good diet but can augment an inadequate one. While supplementation offers a practical means of ensuring adequate intake of essential nutrients, due care must be exercised in choosing the level and type of supplements. The general multivitamin mineral supplements are usually one-a-day pills that contain carefully graded amounts of nutrients and may serve as an 'insurance policy', while the single vitamin and mineral supplements are normally designed for specific health conditions. These require expert advice and should only be taken in consultation with a dietary therapist or a professional nutritional counsellor. Temptation to take higher than stated doses should be resisted as it is possible, in extreme cases, to overdose on certain vitamins and minerals.

However, it is useful to be aware of the different types of nutrients, the elements of a well-balanced diet and any different supplement regimes, so that we can make the right choices. In the subsequent chapters of this book we shall examine the different physical types and lifestyles, and point out where and how to use dietary supplements. Particular attention will be paid to the special needs of children, pregnant and nursing mothers, the elderly and those under stress – the groups most likely to require supplementation for good health and not just the absence of disease.

11

2

Fight Your Way to Health

Man by his habits sets into motion those agencies which eventually destroy him.

Pythagoras

'LIFE BEGINS AT FORTY.' We say it, but hardly ever mean it. Deep down, we think 'I am getting old – I'm over the hill now.'

But have you ever wondered why some fifty-year-olds look and act like forty-year-olds, while others look sixty-five – or older? A factor that determines how we feel, think and look lies in the state of our immune system. In it lie many of the secrets of health, vitality and consequently longevity.

Very simply, the immune system is a personal fighting force that protects the body from attack by bacteria, viruses and other potentially harmful organisms. Further, the immune system helps clear the 'rubbish' that accumulates in our bodies, disposing of dead cells and foreign organisms. Jennifer Meek, author of *Immune Power*, aptly describes it as 'an impressive set up . . . a personal Ministry of Defence and Refuse Disposal Department rolled into one.'

A pristine immune system will ensure that you enjoy optimum health, while an immune system that is 'out of joint' will leave you much more prone to attack by disease-causing organisms, radiation or chemicals. We tend to take good health for granted, little realizing that it is largely thanks to our immune system being on guard twenty-four hours a day.

Ageing
When we are young, our immune system is at its peak to enable us to resist the onslaught of disease. As we get older, we become

12

increasingly prone to degenerative diseases and so at this stage it becomes all the more important to ensure that the immune system is operating at its optimum. Ageing, therefore, is not as inevitable as we normally perceive it to be. Senility and death at around seventy is not a foregone conclusion and we do have some control over the rate at which we age.

Vitality

A well-tuned immune system ensures that we benefit from greater energy. When the immune system is not functioning correctly or is overworked it snatches away some micronutrients and then creates an imbalance in the body's digestive system. This compounds the problem and the body becomes even more prone to diseases. So a good nutrient intake is absolutely essential.

Low Resistance to Disease

An impaired immune system is unable to fight disease. We must therefore keep it well furnished and maintained in order to remain free of infection.

SO WHAT IS THE IMMUNE SYSTEM?

The human body is equipped with a system of defence against disease, and consequently has the the ability to heal itself. When stimulated by disease-causing substances, the immune system is spurred into action. This is sometimes called the *adaptive response*.

As soon as the system encounters a germ or a bug that it perceives as foreign, specialized cells set about fighting to get rid of it. Indeed, the system is so sophisticated that it can actually remember the foreign organism once encountered and is able to respond much quicker in getting rid of it the next time. This is called *acquired immunity*.

Vaccination is an artificial way of acquiring immunity. A small amount of treated or dead organism is injected into the body in a vaccine. As the organism is already treated or dead, there is no danger of acquiring the disease, but, as soon as the body's defence force encounters it, it is put on red alert, fights it, and makes the necessary antibodies. It will also remember how to get rid of it should it encounter a similar organism in the future. So, should one become infected with an active live organism of the same kind (say of smallpox or cholera), the immune system is already aware of its response and will lose no time in preparing antibodies before the foreign organism has had a chance to cause disease.

The thymus gland is the computer database that stores all this information and informs the relevant member of the immune micromilitia when to commence attack, and equally when not to attack in the case of harmless foreign organisms.

As with any sophisticated system, the consequences are serious when it malfunctions. It is therefore important to ensure that the system is properly maintained and not misused. Sometimes the system becomes overactive due to a malfunction and starts attacking harmless foreign substances. Hayfever is a good example of such a malfunction. Normally pollen is a harmless substance and yet some people react violently to it. The reason for this is that the immune system is attacking the harmless pollen particles and releasing a substance called histamine, which results in the familiar pouring out of fluids from the nose and eyes as the body attempts to wash away the 'invader'.

At other times the immune system can go horribly wrong and actually starts attacking the body's own cells. Rheumatoid arthritis is an example of such a malfunction. This is called 'auto-immunity', and diseases caused by such a malfunction are called 'auto-immune diseases'. A transplant can also cause problems, as the immune system rejects the 'foreign' heart or kidney and begins to attack it. In such cases drugs have to be administered to suppress the immune system.

Keeping the Balance

It is important, then, to keep the immune system in a state of balance. Just as a weakened immune system can cause problems so can an overactive one. Indeed, balance is fundamental to good health. Incidences of cancer, auto-immune diseases and immune-related diseases are on the increase. There is a direct correlation here with our lifestyle. Within a very short span of time, we have managed to upset the balance of nature – environmental pollution, the depletion of the ozone layer, pesticides and CFCs are not just buzz words on the agenda of the Green Party and the Greenpeace brigade, but have a lot to answer for in upsetting the finely tuned immune function.

Modern culture has put an additional pressure on the body's immune system. The human body is remarkably adaptable in its quest for survival, but it needs *time* to change, and the pace of change in our environment has overtaken the body's ability to offer the necessary adaptive response. The immune system is overworked and does not always know how to respond to the array of new enemies it now encounters.

If the system cannot eliminate and detoxify a foreign organism, the body is obliged to store it somewhere. The liver, bones and even the brain can become a repository for the waste of dangerous matter. If you add to this the fact that due to modern farming methods our food is robbed of the very nutrients needed to maintain the immune system at its peak, you can understand the surge in the incidence of so-called 'diseases of civilization'.

How Does it Work?

The human immune system is contained in the bloodstream. Our white blood cells carry the combatants through our bloodstream to defend us against attacks from germs, bacteria and viruses. These combatants are broken down into sub-classes based upon their specific abilities and responsibilities in the body's defensive arsenal. T-lymphocytes, or T-cells, for example, engage in hand-to-hand combat with viral invaders. B-lymphocytes secrete highly effective antibodies which are immune-defensive proteins.

If there is a breakdown in these various components of the immune system, the body's ability to fight disease is severely impaired. Individuals whose immune systems are compromised can no longer take that protection for granted and have to endure recurring flu, colds, chronic fatigue and other health problems. However, as long as the immune system is working correctly, at best we are able to avoid the symptoms of illnesses, and at worst the body is able to raise an army quickly to fight disease. For example, a healthy immune system helps destroy cancer cells as they occur and we are therefore able to keep these cells under control.

Nowadays, more than ever before, our immune system is under siege. Firstly there is an increasing array of viruses, some of which can be life threatening, and there are also the more serious viral infections such as herpes, hepatitis and, of course, the Acquired Immune Deficiency Syndrome (AIDS).

The horrific effects of AIDS are essentially due to the severe impairment of the immune system. The Syndrome is caused by the HIV virus (human immune deficiency virus) which breeds inside our white cells and attacks from within, thus severely paralysing our immune system. The victim ultimately dies of common infections and pneumonia, which would otherwise have been effectively dealt with by the immune system.

WHY DOES OUR IMMUNE SYSTEM BECOME WEAK?

You might be surprised to learn that one of the chief culprits is oxygen. Yes, oxygen – the very substance that is essential to life itself. Everyone needs oxygen to stay alive and yet it can also be hazardous to health.

There are two faces to oxygen: the good and the bad. All living things that use oxygen produce what are known as 'free radicals'. If these free radicals are left unchecked they can be harmful to our immune system and do untold damage to our bodies. Free radicals are the cause of rusting iron, hardened rubber and wrinkled skin. They are formed when cells use oxygen. For the process, they produce unstable molecules that lack an electron. Molecules are stable only when they are electronically balanced – free radicals are unstable oxygen molecules.

What Are Free Radicals?

During the process of releasing energy from food, water is generated as a harmless end product. However, sometimes, some of the oxygen that would become water, combines instead with errant electrons to make oxygen free radicals. It is these oxygen free radicals that threaten the cell – if they surge out of control.

Free radicals are created every minute we are alive. The good news is that they are largely held in check by the body's own army of antioxidants. As long as these reactions are kept under control by the body's militia – the antioxidants – we remain healthy. However, if we begin to make too many free radicals, there is a risk of damaging the immune system and developing chronic diseases.

The immune system needs free radicals in small amounts to destroy disease-causing bacteria. But on the other hand these free radicals are electronically unbalanced molecules which will react with and consequently damage surrounding body tissue in an attempt to regain stability. This is because they have a stray or unpaired electron. To recover its stability, the free radical must react with another agent carrying an unpaired electron. When these stray electrons snatch hydrogen atoms from important biological molecules – including fatty acids, proteins and DNA – they set off a chain reaction because the robbed molecule itself becomes a free radical and will try to snatch replacement hydrogen atoms from neighbouring molecules. This chain reaction can damage DNA and cell membranes. Damaged lipids contribute to clogging up the arteries and causing the death of cells in arterial walls, thereby causing heart disease. Damaged DNA may also increase the risk of cancer. Unchecked free radicals are thought to be the most common cause of mutations and cancers, memory loss and senility, auto-immune diseases, ageing and wrinkles.

The polyunsaturated fats that make up the body cell walls are particularly sensitive to free radical attack. When free radicals attack these fats, they become rancid (oxidized) and are structurally damaged. Dr Sharon in his book *The Complete Guide to Nutrition* writes,

> Most free radicals in the body are formed when unsaturated fats auto-oxidize. This process is very similar to what happens when oily rags or rags used to clean oil-based paint from brushes spontaneously catch fire. The unsaturated fatty acids in oil or paint readily react with oxygen in the air, the reaction releases energy as heat and the temperature of the rag eventually reaches ignition point.

The same type of reaction takes place in the human body. It takes just one free radical to oxidize one molecule of unsaturated fat in order for a chain reaction to start. As each molecule of fat is oxidized, another free radical is released which oxidizes another molecule of fat and so on. So a single free radical can oxidize millions of fat molecules. Of course, the body does not ignite like a pile of rags because it contains so much water, but that does not mean that it is not being damaged.

Outside Factors

In addition to the body's normal production of free radicals, there are outside factors that can contribute to our free radical burden. These include:

- Excessive exposure to X-rays.
- Radioactive contamination.
- Pesticides, industrial solvents and CFCs.
- Pollution.

- Smoking – passive and active.

Thus we are constantly being exposed to free radical attack, not just on the X-ray table but also from food, water, cosmetics, drugs, cigarette smoke and the many other pollutants of modern living. Whether from outside or generated in the body, free radicals can be hazardous to human health and it is important to neutralize them before they do any damage.

Protection from Free Radicals

Our protection from free radicals comes from specific micronutrients called antioxidants. An antioxidant is a substance that can protect foods – especially fats and oils – from oxidation, from going rancid. Just as its name suggests, it discourages substances from being oxidized in the body by preventing oxygen from combining with other substances. In this way, it curbs the chain reaction. The nutrients that are commonly thought of as our first line of defence against free radical attack are vitamins C, E, beta carotene and selenium.

In September 1991 the UK Ministry of Agriculture, Fisheries and Food launched a £1.65 million research programme to find out how antioxidant nutrients can protect against various illnesses, such as heart disease, certain cancers and rheumatoid arthritis. This research is part of a larger European initiative investigating the role of antioxidants. Altogether the eating habits of half a million people will be investigated. On the basis of the knowledge to date, it is expected that a high intake of antioxidant-rich foods (fruits, vegetables and vegetable oils) will be shown to protect against cancers of the lung, stomach, large bowel and oesophagus.

According to the *New Scientist* (30th November 1991):

> The British researchers expect the European study to underscore the long supposed benefits of vitamins found in fruits and vegetables. The most effective antioxidant nutrients appear to be vitamins C, E and beta carotene.

What are Antioxidants?

Free radicals have earned themselves the reputation of being the 'bad guys' in the human immune system but, as we have seen, they are necessary to human life and only become hazardous when present in excess. The human body, marvel that it is, has a defence system which in a healthy body can keep free radicals in check – although over the age of forty even this becomes less efficient. As we have seen, the defences against free radicals are antioxidants, since they mop up excess free radicals by binding to them and thus neutralizing their potentially damaging effects.

Commonly recognized antioxidants are vitamins C and E, plus beta carotene (one of the carotenoids), and the minerals selenium and zinc.

Since vitamins and minerals cannot be produced by the body itself and must therefore come from the diet, it is easy to see the correlation between nutrition and a healthy immune system. If your diet is lacking in any of the antioxidants, how can your body deal with the hazard of excess free radicals?

Fighting Free Radicals with Food

We have already established that the nutrients we take in can have a profound effect on how well or badly the immune system functions. It must be stressed that all nutrients are important, but there are specific dietary aspects that must be considered when eating to boost the immune system. The consumption of fats and cholesterol, protein intake, and dietary fibre are important if we are to eat defensively.

(Drugs, smoking and alcohol can all impair the immune system – a puff of cigarette smoke can contain up to 100 trillion free radicals!).

A great deal of attention has recently focused upon the importance of vitamins to health. Let's now take a closer look at those nutrients which are antioxidants. Several vitamins and minerals have antioxidant properties either as part of an antioxidant enzyme system or individually. The trace minerals selenium, copper and manganese combine with an enzyme to destroy free radicals. On the other hand, Vitamins E, C, A, B6 and beta carotene and the mineral zinc function independently of enzymes to inactivate free radicals.

Vitamin C
Vitamin C plays a valuable role in numerous body functions, but here we shall concentrate specifically on its role as an antioxidant. Vitamin C (ascorbate) is perhaps one of the most researched of the

antioxidant substances. Ascorbate is soluble in water and provides antioxidant protection for the watery compartments of our cells, tissues and organs. Our bodies cannot make our own ascorbate so we are dependent upon food sources for this vital nutrient. It is worth knowing that bioflavonoids sometimes occur alongside ascorbate and that they also have antioxidant properties.

Dr Mark Levine of the National Institute of Health in the US has studied the effects of vitamin C on white blood cells. His work has shown that vitamin C is critical to the disease-fighting ability of the white blood cells. Dr Linus Pauling found that the level of vitamin C in the white blood cells is closely related to the body's ability to combat infection – in effect, it plays an important part in boosting the immune system.

Vitamin C is found in citrus fruit, green vegetables, potatoes and fruit juice, so a sufficient consumption of these foods will go a long way to ensuring we get an adequate supply of the vitamin. Several case control studies suggest that consumption of vitamin C-rich foods is associated with a lower risk of some cancers.

Vitamin E

It is astonishing, given the depth of research into this vitamin, that it was only in 1991 that a recommended daily intake of this nutrient was established.

Alpha tocopherol, to give vitamin E its other name, is a powerful nutrient which, in common with many others, plays a crucial role in overall health. As an enzyme-independent antioxidant, alpha tocopherol has a very powerful antioxidant effect on the body, particularly protecting the lipids in cell walls (lipids are particularly susceptible to oxidation by free radicals).

Vitamin E can act to reduce the oxygen requirement of muscles and so increase exercise capacity. As an antioxidant, it has a myriad of vital functions. It stabilizes membranes and protects them against free radical damage, protects the eyes, skin, liver, breast and calf muscle tissues, prevents tumour growth (associated with cancer), protects the lungs from oxidative damage (caused by air pollutants), and protects and increases the body's store of vitamin A. It also protects against the oxidation of polyunsaturated fatty acids (PUFAs) by peroxides, superoxides and other free radicals.

Vitamin E is enhanced by other antioxidants, such as vitamin C and the mineral selenium. Quantities of vitamin E are expressed in either of two ways – by weight (mg) or as a biological activity (i.u). Although there is no definitive recommendation on vitamin

E intake, the COMA Report of 1991 gives several guidelines (see p. 132).

Foods rich in vitamin E include oils (for example, wheatgerm, safflower, sunflower, soyabean), nuts and seeds, wheatgerm, asparagus, spinach, broccoli, butter, bananas and strawberries.

Vitamin A

Studies on laboratory animals are mounting up to show that vitamin A is an anticarcinogenic by maintaining healthy epithelium, but care has to be taken with this vitamin since it can be toxic if taken in too great a quantity.

The first fat-soluble vitamin to be identified, vitamin A is the general name for a group of substances which include retinol, retinal and the carotenoids. The active forms of vitamin A are found in animal tissue; the provitarium (or precursor) form is found in dark green and also orange vegetables and fruits (for example, beta carotene). The carotene precursors of vitamin A need bile and fats to be present in the intestines in order to be absorbed, whereas the active preformed vitamin A is not as fat dependent and as such is better absorbed.

Although this vitamin is stable to light and heat, it is destroyed by the ultra-violet rays of the sun and by oxidation. The presence of vitamin E is therefore valuable, since it sacrifices itself to protect vitamin A (see p. 20, vitamin E).

Vitamin A is found in eggs, milk, lamb's liver, halibut liver oil, cod liver oil, dairy products, pig's kidney, carrots, beef, mackerel and canned sardines.

Zinc

Zinc is found in alpha-macroglobulin (an important protein in the body's immune system), so it stands to reason that a shortage of this mineral will severely affect the immune system. What's more, zinc can help to clear certain toxic metals from the body (for instance, cadmium and lead – present in car exhaust fumes). Zinc is also essential for normal cell division and function so, in addition to its antioxidant activities, it also plays a part in protecting the cells. In fact, zinc functions in more enzymatic reactions than any other trace mineral.

Zinc is present in dairy products, beef, chicken, white fish and bread. It is an all-round valuable nutrient, so make sure your intake is satisfactory. A common sign of zinc deficiency is white marks on the fingernails.

Beta Carotene

As explained in the section on vitamin A, beta carotene is the precursor to vitamin A and therefore functions in a different way – it has to be converted in to vitamin A before it can be used. Beta carotene is nevertheless a powerful destroyer of free radicals so it is important to ensure an adequate intake.

Studies have shown that smokers and heavy drinkers have very low levels of beta carotene. Studies have also revealed that patients with certain cancers (colon, lung, skin, mouth) have previously eaten less beta carotene-rich diets than the healthy controls. Trials investigating beta carotene's use as an actual treatment for cancer have yet to be carried out, but the evidence suggests it can help prevent cancers in its role as a destroyer of free radicals.

You will find beta carotene in spinach, carrots, kale, broccoli, peaches and apricots – the orange and green vegetables and fruit.

Dosage

Before you start taking copious amounts of the antioxidant nutrients above the RDA level, it is worth stopping a moment. The immune system can be both strengthened and weakened by dietary intake of nutrients. Optimal (the recommended) intake of vitamins A, C and E and the mineral zinc will strengthen the immune system, increasing resistance to colds and more serious infections, but larger daily doses actually suppress the immune system. This is because the immune system includes several feedback mechanisms which recognize higher than required intakes. Consequently the system 'slows down', to cope with the increased intake.

THE DIET/HEALTH CONNECTION

As we have seen, scientists have noted the correlation between health and specific types of diet. For example, in the US and UK, deaths from heart disease are the highest in the world. The diets of these two countries are highly refined and loaded with processed and high fat foods, such as burgers, chips, dairy produce, and red meat. Also, consumption of fresh fruit and vegetables in these countries is noticeably lower per capita than elsewhere in the world. Mediterranean people enjoy pasta, rich cheeses, sauces and red meat, yet whilst in some cases they may be just as overweight as their British and American counterparts, they have a significantly low rate of heart disease probably because of their high consumption of fresh fruit and vegetables.

In November 1991 a group of European scientists began the mammoth task of monitoring the eating habits of around half a million people. The results will not be forthcoming until the end of the century but will be worth waiting for. Meanwhile, the International Agency for Research on Cancer is currently carrying out a four-year study at Lyons in France, to establish the effects of diet on cancers of the lung, colon, prostate, stomach and breast. Provided sponsoring continues after this initial period, research will continue into the connection between diet and the rarer forms of cancer.

From the body of research on the individual antioxidant nutrients, vitamins A, C and E, and the mineral zinc, it is safe to emphasize their importance in boosting the immune system – and therefore in protecting yourself against heart disease and cancer. However, it must also be said that simply taking supplements will not make up for eating fatty foods, smoking and not taking exercise – the whole health perspective has to be taken into account. Antioxidants probably act by protecting the delicate living cells of coronary (and other) blood vessels from damage by free radicals, which may pave the way for deposition of cholesterol and thrombus, thus narrowing these important arteries. When a diseased and narrow artery becomes totally blocked by a clot, the portion of heart muscle dependent on that artery dies (myocardial infarction).

Beauty

Over the last decade, experts have acknowledged the role of free radicals in the ageing process. The trouble starts when the body slows its free radical surveillance under the influence of such oxygenators as sunlight, stress, cigarette smoke, smog and certain medications (particularly antibiotics). You can tell that the skin cells are losing the ageing war when wrinkles deepen, the skin sags, age spots darken and skin cancers appear.

While using sunscreens, moisturizers and night treatments, particularly those containing antioxidants such as tocopherol, beta carotene and selenium, can help, we all know the truth of the statement 'beauty comes from within'. An unhealthy diet will quickly show itself in poor skin and hair, while an effective intake of antioxidants will help to destroy the free radicals responsible for the ageing process.

So enjoy your fresh fruit and vegetables in the knowledge that not only are you taking a step towards a healthier immune system – you will also look better.

An Efficient Immune System will
- Decrease the severity of infections
- Reduce the likelihood of catching colds, flu and other infections
- Maximize the destruction of cancer cells
- Reduce the chances of auto-immune diseases
- Increase energy levels by dispersing the accumulation of toxic chemicals that sap vitality
- Protect the body from radiation and other pollutants in the environment
- Slow the ageing process

Some Common Immune-related Diseases
- AIDS – Acquired Immune Deficiency Syndrome.
- Cancer and Tumours
- Rheumatoid Arthritis
- Allergies
- Food Sensitivity

The Attack on the Immune System
- Infections
- Negative Mental Attitude
- Stress
- Malnutrition
- Radiation
- Lack of Exercise
- Chemicals

Symptoms of an Impaired Immune System
- Indigestion
- Swollen and painful glands
- Loss of smell, mucus, difficulty in breathing
- Hair loss and dull hair
- Wrinkled and dry skin
- Stiff and swollen joints
- Poor concentration, lack of interest, lethargy
- Depression, irritability

NUTRIENTS THAT HELP THE IMMUNE SYSTEM

Vitamin A and Beta Carotene
- Responsible for growth and maintaining an active thymus, and hence a strong immune system.

- Powerful antivirals – important for strong linings in areas of special risk, such as the gut and the respiratory system.

Vitamin C
- Antiviral.
- Boosts production of prostaglandin E and increases production of T-Lymphocytes.
- Increases production of interferon.
- Detoxifies many bacterial toxins.
- Improves the performance of antibiotics.

Vitamin E
- Necessary for normal antibody response.
- Neutralizes free radicals.
- Works with other nutrients to improve resistance to infections.
- Protects against air pollution.

Iron
- Essential for antibody production.
- Required for the enzyme 'myeloperoxide' used in the formation of white blood cells. (The enzyme myeloperoxide is needed by the white blood cells (neutrophils or polymorphs) in their function of attacking foreign organisms.)

Selenium
- A good antioxidant – works with vitamin E.
- Protects against cancer-causing substances.
- Is used in antibody production.
- Without it, white cells seem to lose their ability to recognize invaders.

Zinc
- Needed for enzymes which destroy cancer cells.
- Thymulin, the hormone necessary for maturation of T-cells, is dependent on zinc.

ANTINUTRIENTS THAT AFFECT THE IMMUNE SYSTEM

Fluoride
- Slows the immune system.
- Reduces the ability of the white cells to destroy foreign cells.

Mercury
- Adversely affects the body's ability to fight infection.
- Adversely affects the body's ability to distinguish between foreign and other organisms.
- Makes antibodies to poison the body's own (white) cells.
- Adversely affects the brain and the nervous system.

Cadmium
- Inhibits the function of some enzymes containing antibodies.

Aluminium
- Interferes with calcium utilization and compromises bone function and immune function.
- Affects haemoglobin production.

ANTIOXIDANT AMINO ACIDS

Some amino acids also have very powerful antioxidant and detoxifying properties. When the body is exposed to toxins it is therefore crucial to have enough antioxidant amino acids in the diet, through food sources and supplementation:

L-Methionine
- A heavy metal detoxifier which lowers excessive levels of lead and copper in the blood, thus counteracting toxicity symptoms.
- It also has the ability to detoxify excess histamine in the body, thus helping to fight allergic conditions.

L-Cysteine
- Active against free radicals because of its chemical structure.
- Helps reduce oxidation in sensitive tissues by sacrificing itself for oxidation first.

Glutathione
- Through its involvement in the body's enzyme system, it protects both the liver and lungs from the effects of car exhaust fumes, and damage to the body from smoking and alcohol abuse.

3

Women's Special Requirements

ONCE UPON A TIME, girls would grow up, marry, and spend the rest of their lives looking after their husband and bringing up a family. Today, women often follow the same path but also hold down a steady job. Some women – the 'superwomen' – hold down a top career job as well as bringing up a family, looking after their husbands, and running the house. Is it any wonder that they can find there just aren't enough hours in the day? With the advent of convenience foods, traditional homecooking has become something of a treat, and saving time in the kitchen in this way inevitably takes its toll on health since convenience foods are often more a chemist's than a cook's concoction.

In many ways a woman's nutritional requirements are higher than a man's, since every month she menstruates and this involves many different bodily functions. An inadequate diet will cause a deficiency of nutrients essential to good health. This will make itself very quickly felt in painful periods and sometimes PMT. Further, when a woman is pregnant a healthy diet is vital if she is to enjoy a healthy pregnancy and give birth to a healthy child. If she then opts to breastfeed her newborn – which is best for her baby – correct nutritional intake is paramount. Later, when her child-bearing years are over and she goes through 'the change', a lack of important nutrients may well cause severe problems in later life.

In this chapter we shall look at the key stages in a woman's life in which correct nutrition, aided by sensible supplementation, will ensure good health.

PRECONCEPTUAL NUTRITION

Research shows that what you eat before conception will have an effect on the child itself. Professor Michael Crawford has undertaken a good deal of research into preconceptual nutrition and its effect on the future child. In 1990 the Institute of Brain Chemistry and Human Nutrition was founded in Hackney, and research carried out there has substantiated findings in Italy, France, Japan, the USA and Canada that poor nutrition during early phase of brain development affects the brain permanently. Studies of over five hundred pregnancies at the Institute have established the clear correlation between the health and nutrition of the mother before conception and the health of her baby. Further, mothers who were deficient in forty-three out of the forty-four nutrients analysed, gave birth to low birthweight babies, and also to babies with a higher incidence of brain disorders. The deficiencies most closely connected with low birthweight are thiamin, pyridoxine, riboflavin, folic acid, chloride and magnesium.

The Institute has also accumulated experimental evidence which implies that arachidonic (AA) and decosahexaenoic (DHA) acids may be beneficial in protecting a premature baby's brain from cerebral palsy and development of spasticity. Formula-fed babies have less plasma AA and DHA than breast-fed babies, and as these acids are specifically used in brain growth the recent reporting that breast-fed babies are more intelligent than those which are formula-fed can be understood. Additional studies in Dallas, USA, have shown formula-fed babies to have poor visual ability and mental performance at eighteen months compared to those who were breast-fed or supplemented with DHA. Attention to nutrition during pregnancy and after the birth is beneficial but cannot rectify the effects of a poor diet prior to conception, so it is important that mothers-to-be pay diligent attention to their diet when planning to start a family.

PAINFUL PERIODS: WHO NEEDS THEM?

Nobody wants painful periods, but unfortunately they are a common fact of life. Not for nothing is menstruation nicknamed 'the curse'. While it is normal for a certain amount of discomfort to arise from uterine contractions, the additional symptoms of headaches, dizziness, nausea, vomiting and fatigue can be a sign of inadequate nutrition and as such can easily be eradicated.

Drug-free relief from *dysmenorrhea* (the medical term for painful periods) is possible by following a wholefood diet, taking regular exercise, and relaxing. Useful supplements include:

- A multivitamin and mineral complex.
- Vitamin C with bioflavonoids.
- Vitamin B complex.
- Iron.
- Calcium and magnesium.
- Evening primrose oil.
- Ginseng (for vitality and energy).
- Royal jelly.

They say that 'every cloud has a silver lining' and this is also true of 'the curse'. Effectively, if menstruation is causing serious health problems you are receiving an alarm call from your body that you haven't been treating it well. It is then up to you to do something to reverse the situation, because nobody *has* to suffer from painful periods.

PREMENSTRUAL TENSION (PMT)

Do You Suffer From PMT?

How do you know if you suffer from PMT? It is quite simple to find out whether PMT is an actuality for you – or an excuse for general grouchiness and bad behaviour! There are four different types of PMT, as recorded by Dr Guy Abraham:

- **PMT A** Anxiety, irritability, mood swings — affects 80 per cent of sufferers.
- **PMT B** Bloating, breast tenderness, abdominal bloating, weight gain, swollen extremities — affects 60 per cent of sufferers.
- **PMT C** Craving carbohydrates (especially chocolate), headaches, fatigue, increased appetite, dizziness and fainting — affects 40 per cent of sufferers.

- **PMT D** Depression,
  insomnia, crying, distress,
  confusion, forgetfulness   affects 20 per cent of sufferers.

Sufferers of PMT A usually experience the symptoms of PMT D as well.

A typical sufferer experiences PMT symptoms for seven to ten days before her period is due, and once her period begins all symptoms abruptly cease. If you don't know already if PMT is a problem for you, keep a note of how you feel during the month, for two months at least. Note when you feel irritable, moody, and so on and at the end of the two months you should be able to see either a clear pattern of symptoms occurring in the run-up to your period, ceasing once menstruation begins (in which case you are suffering from PMT), or that your symptoms are scattered throughout the month – in which case it would be necessary to look at other elements in your life to determine why your health is below par.

If PMT is your problem, you will undoubtedly want to do something to free yourself from what seems to be a curse which ruins two weeks out of every four – and your partner and family, as well as work colleagues, will be just as keen for you to rout the problems of PMT. After all, it is not just you who suffers – everyone around you suffers the repercussions too!

Causes of PMT

Investigation of PMT sufferers has disclosed a common shortage of the hormone progesterone. Treatment of PMT has consequently been via prescription of progesterone supplements, which normally ease the symptoms but rarely eradicate them.

Many women have been prescribed pyridoxine (vitamin B6) to ease PMT. This is because B6 is required in the production of dopamine and serotonin, compounds which have a calming effect. B6 can, therefore, help to keep you on an even keel emotionally. Further, B6 can affect prolactin which, in excess, is responsible for many PMT symptoms, typically weight gain, breast tenderness, fluid retention, depression and irritability. Prolactin affects the quantities of oestrogen and progesterone present during each cycle, which must be in the right balance if the body is to function correctly.

Whilst this does provide relief in many cases, it is not the sole solution for PMT.

Women taking evening primrose oil (EPO) supplements for a variety of health complaints (acne, arthritis, high blood pressure) have found, as a side effect, that their PMT symptoms either vanish or are substantially relieved.

Many studies are now showing that PMT is caused by:

- A hormonal imbalance.
- A defect in essential fatty acid (EFA) metabolism.

Attention to both factors will therefore be necessary in any successful treatment of PMT.

Essential Fatty Acids (EFAs) and PMT

Essential fatty acids are sometimes referred to as vitamin F. So the fact that they have vitamin status tells us that these nutrients are necessary for healthy body functioning yet cannot be manufactured by the body itself. An inadequate amount of particular EFAs may, depending on the type of diet consumed, lead to unchecked levels of cholesterol and all the problems which that brings. EFAs are found in vegetable oils, fish and, to a much smaller degree, in animal fats.

Polyunsaturates are essential fatty acids and most of us are aware of their role in good cardiovascular health – and may consequently have switched from eating butter to one of the vegetable oil-based margarines. Unfortunately, given the nature of linoleic acid (the key EFA), the body may not be able to derive full benefit from polyunsaturates.

Linoleic acid has to be converted into prostaglandin E1 to be of benefit to us, and as this conversion is affected by many factors it may be very inefficient.

Evening Primrose Oil

Commonly known as 'King's Cure All' in centuries past, the oil of the evening primrose is truly remarkable in its widely beneficial effects on human health, but here we shall concentrate on its relevance to the relief of PMT (for more on EPO see Chapter 6). The end-product of linoleic acid, PGE1, is vital for hormonal balance, and a lack of PGE1 produces the symptoms of PMT. A lack of pyridoxine (vitamin B6) has long been linked to PMT, and it is interesting to note that this is one of the nutrients whose presence is necessary for the conversion of GLA to PGE1. Treatment of PMT with B6 would therefore improve matters, where a deficiency existed, but by itself would not eliminate PMT.

Other nutrients which play a vital role in PGE1 conversion are vitamins C and E, and the minerals zinc and selenium (see diagram on p. 69).

PMT Fighters

We can now draw up a 'shopping list' of nutrients which protect against PMT:

- Evening Primrose Oil.
- Vitamin E.
- Vitamin C (ascorbic acid).
- Zinc.
- Selenium.
- Vitamin B6 (pyridoxine).
- Magnesium.
- Calcium.

Studies have shown that treatment with evening primrose oil can eradicate PMT altogether, and at the very least greatly reduce its unpleasant symptoms in ninety-five per cent of users.

Diet Against PMT

Avoid refined foods, alcohol and fats. Increase intake of wholefoods, sugar, white meat, fish, complex carbohydrates, fresh fruit and vegetables. (It would be best to give up smoking, too.)

THE MENOPAUSE

The menopause usually starts between the ages of forty-five and fifty-five and can last for one year or eleven, although the average duration is five years.

The first sign for most women that they have entered the menopause is a sudden irregularity of the menstrual flow. At the same time, a reduced level of the female hormones, oestrogen and progesterone, triggers other symptoms, including hot flushes, irritability, mood swings, depression, weight increase, fluid retention, vaginal dryness, skin and hair changes, sleep problems and loss of libido. Added to all that, osteoporosis (see below) is an increasing health problem for women in their menopausal years.

Obviously the symptoms of the menopause affect many different areas of the body, and therefore a variety of supplements is required to ease the situation. It should not be forgotten though that, in addition to good nutrition, an overall healthy lifestyle should be adopted for a sense of well-being: this includes regular exercise, relaxation, and a positive attitude to greet this new era in your life. With the menopause a woman reaches the end of her child-bearing years, not the end of her ability for creativity in other areas and the capacity to enjoy life to the full. Indeed, studies have shown that career women or those with an active home-life suffer from menopausal problems less frequently than those with little to occupy them.

Most of the menopausal symptoms are related to falling oestrogen levels which occur in all women undergoing the change, and one possible reason for the reduced symptoms in a busy women could be that a positive and cheerful attitude may modify the effect of reduced oestrogen levels.

Make Life Easy

The menopause, like puberty, is a time of transition and the body needs all the help it can get to effect this transition as smoothly as possible. From a general viewpoint this means:

- No smoking.
- As little refined food as possible.
- No alcohol.
- Eat as much fresh fruit and vegetables as you can (the World Health Organization recommends a pound a day).
- Eat fish, nuts (not the roasted, salted kind!).
- Eat wholemeal bread.
- Keep consumption of fats as low as possible.

Oestrogen

Many of the symptoms associated with the menopause are the result of decreasing levels of oestrogen – part of the body's overall cutting-back on hormone production. When hormone levels drop drastically the body is 'in shock', if you like, at the sudden change, and symptoms are pronounced. It helps, therefore, to ingest oestrogen so that the decrease is gradual rather than sudden. For this reason women are commonly prescribed hormone replacement therapy (HRT) which consists of drug treatment.

HRT solves the problems of hot flushes and vaginal dryness almost immediately, and it is thought to reduce the risk of osteoporosis by as much as fifty per cent over five to six years. But there are drawbacks. Menstruation returns on a regular basis and with it the symptoms of PMT. Research has also suggested that HRT may increase the risk of breast cancer and thrombosis – but research is not certain on this point as yet. However, if you are in a high risk group of osteoporosis and neither you nor your family has a history of breast cancer or thrombosis, it may be beneficial to undergo HRT. Your doctor should be able to explain the pros and cons to you.

There are, however, other ways of obtaining oestrogen-like substances from herbs, roots and fruits. Amongst many others, these include:

- Ginseng.
- Liquorice root.
- Elder.

- Wild yam.
- Lady's slipper.
- Cucumber.

The herbs can be bought from a health food store and made into herbal tea. Alternatively, some of the herbs and roots are available in capsule form which you may prefer. Bear in mind, though, that herbs were the first medicine known to mankind. They are not to be treated lightly, and care should be taken in their use. You will be well advised to consult a herbalist.

Sleep Easy

Continued insomnia can drive a person to distraction – or to sleeping pills. Neither cures the problem so both should be avoided!

There are several herbal sleep-inducing remedies available now.

These formulations combine herbs such as valerian or skullcap. Valerian is also beneficial for headaches and indigestion. As far as food goes, complex carbohydrates (for example, wholemeal bread, brown rice and other grains) are the key to promoting relaxation and thus sleep.

Make sure you eat food containing complex carbohydrates like wholemeal bread and crackers which do not have salt liberally sprinkled all over them! Complex carbohydrate foods keep the blood sugar on an even keel (low blood sugar makes you weak and edgy) and allow the brain to utilize the amino acid, tryptophan. Tryptophan is used by the brain to create serotonin which is a calming agent. A high protein intake interferes with serotonin, so high protein foods should be avoided. Magnesium also helps to keep you calm so a supplement of this mineral can also help.

Osteoporosis

As a woman ages her skeleton loses its calcium content with the result that it becomes brittle – this condition is osteoporosis. A safeguard is to ensure that calcium levels are kept high throughout life so that upon approaching the menopause the skeleton is in good, strong order. However, once having reached the menopause a calcium supplement is advisable. These supplements will include magnesium without which calcium cannot be absorbed by the body. Calcium-rich foods include dairy products, but gorging on cheese, butter, milk and yoghourt is not a good idea as these are mucus-forming and high in animal fats.

Hot Flushes

Unfortunately, the cause of hot flushes has not as yet been established. Several theories exist but none is yet definitive. The important factor is that, whilst being a major discomfort, hot flushes are not life-threatening and will pass with the menopause.

The elements of hot flushes – raised temperature and expanded capillaries – can be relieved with supplements. Vitamin E has been used successfully to treat hot flushes for some time, and vitamin E also works towards a good complexion, improving the circulation, and much more. Oestrogen depletes vitamin E so, if you are taking hormones or oestrogen-rich herbs, vitamin E is even more worthwhile. Flushes are the result of the blood vessels expanding, so with recurrent flushes the capillary walls are constantly expanding and contracting. To prevent damage to the capillary walls vitamin C with bioflavonoids can be taken, a treatment which has been shown to be effective in the treatment of hot flushes.

Diet for the Menopause

A wholefood diet which eliminates processed foods is essential during the menopause because there are a number of nutrients which act directly upon the symptoms and can go a long way towards relieving them.

A wholefood diet is one which contains complete carbohydrates. The extra bulk provided by the fibre keeps bowels healthy by ensuring all waste is eliminated (constipation is no longer a problem), and, of course, wholefoods are more filling than their refined counterparts because of their extra bulk.

Summary
- Add fibre, from cereals, wholegrain bread, fresh fruit and vegetables.
- Reduce caffeine intake, since this is a stimulant and can exacerbate hot flushes.
- Reduce salt and saturated fat intake, since these increase the risk of water retention and heart disease (see Chapter 4).
- Avoid excessive alcohol since it can affect nutrient absorption and can cause high blood pressure. It may also act as a depressant, and aggravate mood changes.
- Follow a wholefood diet.
- Eat oily fish both for the protein content and for the supply of fish oils which are beneficial to heart health.

Supplements for the Menopause

In order to ensure that the body's biochemical needs are being met it is wise to consider supplementing a wholefood diet with dietary supplements. There are certain conditions – menopause being one of them – that make extra demands upon the body. The following supplements are recommended:

- A good time-release, multivitamin and mineral supplement – this will improve your general health and assist the function of other nutrients to combat specific symptoms.
- Vitamin E – highly effective in relieving flushes. This has to be taken for three to four months for it to be effective.
- Vitamin C with bioflavonoids – an antistress vitamin to combat the effects of excess wear and tear, both mental and physical.
- A vitamin B complex supplement – in addition to being an antistress vitamin, the B-complex also facilitates effective function of vitamin E.
- Calcium (also a protection against osteoporosis).
- Magnesium.
- Evening primrose oil – helps regulate hormonal imbalances, and ensures the adequate manufacture of essential prostaglandins.
- Zinc.

PREGNANCY AND BREASTFEEDING

It goes without saying that pregnancy makes great demands on a woman's body. During this time, good nutrition is essential for the health of both mother and baby.

It is a great temptation to rely on heavily on widely available convenience foods, many of which are highly processed and full of numerous additives and preservatives. As a result, many people fall into the habit of eating a poorly balanced diet – not enough fibre, too much fat, too much sugar and salt, and not enough fresh fruit and vegetables – exactly the kind of diet which all of us, but particularly pregnant women, should try to avoid.

A poorly balanced diet will eventually leave the mother in short supply of essential nutrients, but this deficiency is doubled during pregnancy since the baby draws reserves from the mother for its own needs, leaving the mother still further depleted of nutrients. If this process is allowed to continue, even the baby will eventually be unable to get enough of the vitamins and minerals it needs, thus impairing his or her health.

The vitamin B complex, vitamins C and E, iron, zinc, manganese, magnesium, chromium and calcium are especially important during pregnancy, but in fact it is worth concentrating on getting *all* the nutrients you need since all will be used to help nourish the growing child.

Diet During Pregnancy

During pregnancy it is important to eat as varied a diet as possible:

- Include plenty of fresh fruit and vegetables for vitamin intake (especially A, C, and E).
- Include protein and fibre from fish, eggs, lean meat, cheese, almonds, lentils, pulses and grains. Protein is essential for the growth and repair of body tissues – of both mother and child. A shortage of protein during pregnancy can lead to toxaemia.
- Steer clear of fats.
- Steer clear of refined sugars and highly processed foods: far from nourishing the body these foods place an extra demand on it.
- Avoid frying and overcooking: grill, poach and steam foods instead.

Morning Sickness

Unfortunately, simply following general guidelines will not necessarily stave off the dreaded morning sickness. Relief can sometimes be obtained by taking ginger (an ancient remedy), and vitamin B6 can also be helpful. Oestrogen is high during pregnancy, and this affects vitamin B6 uptake. Use of the contraceptive pill also depletes B6 and if a woman has been taking the pill over a considerable time before deciding to start a family, shortage of this vitamin could have steadily built up.

Nausea and persistent vomiting are possible signs of magnesium deficiency, and other symptoms include swollen gums, hair loss, upset tummy, muscle 'shakes' and lack of appetite). Do ensure that you are getting enough of this valuable mineral.

Other Beneficial Supplements for Pregnancy

Vitamin C with bioflavonoids will, amongst other benefits, strengthen the capillary walls and this may help guard against varicose veins. Calcium and magnesium supplements will be necessary if leg cramps occur, whilst zinc may help counteract stretch marks. Alternatively, vitamin E massaged into the skin has received favourable reports for combating stretch marks. Generally, a good multivitamin/mineral taken throughout pregnancy should ensure good health for both mother and child.

IS BREAST BEST?

The answer is Yes. We stated earlier that essential fatty acids are found in evening primrose, borage, and human milk. Essential fatty acids protect the body and are vital for many body functions. In addition, breast milk contains antibodies which are passed from mother to baby. Recent research shows that omega-3s (a family of essential fats) are also present in human milk but not in formula milk. So what you have in breast milk is something far more complicated than Man in his egotistical way believes can be all too easily emulated. Human milk is a veritable potion of goodness which nurtures the growing infant not only by nourishing but also, unlike formula milk, by building up the infant's bodily mechanisms. Unless you are simply not producing milk, the question of whether to go for breast or bottle should be immaterial if the baby's needs are to be taken into consideration.

The nutritional needs of a lactating mother are even higher than during pregnancy, particularly for vitamins, calcium, zinc, magnesium and other minerals. To ensure sufficient of the necessary nutrients, the breastfeeding mother should aim to eat a wide variety of foods in as close to their natural state as possible.

Sometimes the baby will be adversely affected by what its mother eats, causing problems such as colic, diarrhoea, constant crying, and skin problems. It really is a matter of experimenting to find out which are the problem foods, but common culprits are dairy products, wheat, citrus fruits, spicy foods, and excessive caffeine intake.

4

Twentieth-century Ailments

It is strange, but true – for truth is always strange
Byron (1788–1823)

T ECHNOLOGICAL INNOVATION and increased affluence, coupled with modern marketing techniques, have all led to major changes in the nutritional composition of our diet. It is estimated that our fat and sugar consumption (per capita) has increased five- to ten-fold over the last two centuries, whilst consumption of cereals and grains has declined substantially. On the scale of human history, these changes represent a dramatic and sudden change in our food supply.

While an increased and easily available supply of food has eliminated starvation and deficiency diseases in most of the developed countries, the long-term health effects of foods rich in fat and sugar have only been identified in the last few decades. The correlation between the establishment of this type of diet and the emergence of the so-called 'diseases of civilization' – such as coronary heart disease, cancer and various bone and joint disorders – has been amply demonstrated.

CANCER

As our knowledge of nutrition becomes more advanced, experts have arrived at a consensus that cancer is a lifestyle disease and can be prevented. The link between diet and cancer has been suspected for some years. This thinking has its roots in the fact that the cure

40

for many other dietary deficient diseases was effected by supplying the missing vital nutrients.

For example, scurvy (a disease whose symptoms include painful joints and weakness) was a common ailment among sailors, explorers and those who lacked fresh foods in their diet for prolonged periods. Although a rare disease today, the period before 1700 was characterized by scurvy epidemics of catastrophic proportions. Vasco da Gama saw over a quarter of his crew of 160 fall prey to terminal scurvy as he sailed round the Cape of Good Hope in 1498.

It was not until the end of the sixteenth century that Sir Richard Hawkins observed during his voyage to the South Seas that the natives used sour oranges and lemons as a cure for scurvy. When tried on his crew, a similar result was noticed. Yet for two hundred years European orthodox medical practitioners refused even to consider this simple treatment. In 1754 Dr James Lind, a surgeon at the Royal Navy Hospital, wrote *A Treatise on the Scurvy* in which he described the preventative and curative effects of oranges and lemons. It was another half-century before European physicians accepted that scurvy was a disease caused by dietary deficiency and were bold enough to prescribe something as simple as lime juice as a cure.

One can perhaps draw parallels with the modern day 'sailor's calamity' of cancer. If Hawkins's anecdotal evidence and Lind's perceptive observations had been heeded, many lives could have been saved. It took more than two hundred years (from 1593 to 1800) to establish that both prevention and cure for scurvy lay not in a sophisticated drug with an unpronounceable name of Latin derivation, but in a simple everyday ingredient in the diet – lime juice! The notion that vitamins and minerals are simply a twentieth-century fad must therefore be discounted.

It is important to understand that the effects of oranges and lemons in the cure for scurvy were known long before vitamin C was singled out as the specific antiscurvy nutrient. It took another hundred years to identify vitamin C as the curative element in limes and oranges and that it was a deficiency in this vitamin that led to scurvy.

Present-day medical research has yet to identify the cause of the dreaded 'lumps' it calls cancer. The orthodox medical response is to physically remove the lump by surgery or radiation, but this cannot guarantee that the lump will not recur nor can it restrict the lump once it has grown beyond a certain point.

As in the case of Hawkins's observations on his voyage to the

South Seas which provided a clue to the nutrition–disease connection, there are a number of observations linking cancer to nutrition. For example, the biochemist, Krebs, confirmed earlier research some sixty years ago that drew our attention to the connection with nutrition.

One such observation is the relatively low incidence of cancer in Utah in the USA. The obvious question which springs to mind is, What is different about Utah from the rest of the USA? A report published by the American Cancer Society (Utah Division) states:

> Utah has an unusual pattern of both new cases of cancer and mortality from cancer. The determinants of this are not clear to the ACS. Certainly a reduced amount of cigarette consumption in the population is one factor. However, this does not fully explain the differences present in sites such as colon, rectum, etc.

The report goes on to compare detailed statistical analysis of Utah cancer with the data for the State of Connecticut, by looking at cancers of the stomach and colon, and acute leukaemia. All this is very scientific and impressive, yet the report does not even hint at the significant differences between the dietary habits of the people in Utah as compared to the people of Connecticut. In their attempts to analyse the different sites of cancer in the body, the researchers appear to have ignored the geography of cancer in the USA – namely, that some states have a significantly low incidence of cancer. Could there be a simple explanation? Perhaps some environmental factors? Pollution? Diet? Maurice Salaman in *Nutrition – The Cancer Answer* writes:

> It has been long established that Seventh Day Adventists have a lower cancer incidence than the general population. This is a widely spread group, every member of which breathes the same air, uses the same soaps – is, in short, subjected to the same environmental hazards as are all of us. There is one outstanding exception: their nutritional preferences, member for member, substantially include whole grains and foods made therefrom.

The question which begs an answer is: is the low cancer rate in Utah related to the high percentage of Seventh Day Adventists in that state?

What is Cancer?

The medical establishment considers all cancers to be different and that each type of cancer is a biologically distinct phenomenon. As there are many types of cancer cells there can be an equal number of treatments. According to experts there are over two hundred types of cancers.

Richard Peto, in *The Causes of Cancer* (Oxford Medical Publications, 1981), writes: 'It makes as little sense to keep together cancers of the lung, stomach and intestine when considering the causes of cancer as to lump together cholera, tuberculosis and syphilis.' By contrast however, the proponents of metabolic approach favour the unitarian thesis that the 'malignant component in all exhibitions of cancers is the same; that this component is not spontaneously created but represents the most primitive cell in the life-cycle – gone awry.' The thesis postulates that the cancer cell is an aberration of a normal cell – one that exists naturally in the body. This cell has malfunctioned and cannot be controlled by the body's immune system.

While experts continue to argue over the complexities of the disease, cancer continues to affect one in three people in Britain. Never mind the cure – even the cause remains an enigma.

The factor which all cancers have in common is the development of mutant (abnormal) cells in the affected part of the body. Inside our bodies, cells are constantly reproducing by dividing themselves into two. Within each cell there is the genetic code which controls the kind of cell that develops and what its function and behaviour will be. Sometimes the cell division produces an abnormal cell which is not coded properly, and when this cell starts to multiply uncontrollably the result is cancer.

As we saw in Chapter 2, it is one of the tasks of the immune function of the body for the white cells to combat and kill abnormal cells. Simply stated, cancers develop when the body's defence militia fails to destroy cells with the wrong genetic code and allows them to multiply unchecked. It so happens that certain mutant cells multiply much faster than others. Some mutant cells may also travel in the body and start other cancers.

Stages in the Development of Cancer
1. Initiation: The cell is first damaged.
2. Promotion: The cell is influenced by other carcinogenic factors.

3. Proliferation: Cells or a group of cells actively mutate to cause a tumour.

Some Facts About Cancer

- It is not a new disease nor is it confined to the West.
- Evidence of bone cancer was found in dinosaur skeletons.
- Hippocrates (460–370 BC) first gave cancer a name, *kariknoma*, which means 'crab'.
- *Cancer* is Latin for 'crab'.
- Lung cancer is the biggest killer, followed by breast cancer, in both the USA and the UK.
- In Australia there is a high incidence of skin cancers.
- There is more stomach cancer in Japan than anywhere else in the world – linked to their high intake of dried salted fish.
- India and France have a high rate of oral cancers.

DIETARY CONSIDERATIONS IN TWENTIETH-CENTURY AILMENTS

It is almost a paradox that the inability to find an effective cure for cancer has instigated much research on its prevention. Of late there has been considerable debate regarding the specific dietary considerations aimed at reducing the risk of developing cancer.

The two main considerations are fat and fibre. A diet high in fat (especially the saturated fats found in fried foods and some vegetable oils), and low in fibre, is thought to be directly linked to the risk of developing several types of cancer (for instance, those of the colon, breast and prostate). If the fibre content of food is increased and the intake of fat decreased the risk is considerably reduced.

At this juncture we can do no better than quote some of the main preventative recommendations of the American Cancer Society:

Avoid Obesity Obese people have an increased risk of cancers of the uterus, stomach, kidney, gall-bladder, colon and breast. A study by the ACS demonstrated that a man forty per cent overweight has thirty-three per cent greater risk of developing cancer, compared to a man who is of normal weight. A woman forty per cent overweight has fifty-five per cent greater risk than a woman who is not overweight.

Eat More High Fibre Foods   High fibre foods are generally rich in nutrients and low in calories and fat. Eating a variety of foods such as fresh fruit, vegetables and whole grains will provide the best source of vitamins and minerals as well as fibrous substances.

Cut Down on Fat Intake   Both saturated and unsaturated fat in excess have been found to promote cancer. Cutting back on fatty foods, fats and oils, also helps to maintain correct body weight as they are the major sources of superfluous calories.

Cut Down on Alcohol   In addition to causing liver cancer, alcohol abuse also increases the risk of cancers of the mouth, larynx and oesophagus. This risk is even greater in alcohol abusers who are also smokers.

Reduce Consumption of Smoked and Salt-Cured and Nitrite-Cured Foods   Nitrates and nitrites are common preservatives used in meats. They are also used to cure or pickle foods. These chemicals can form nitrosamines which in turn are carcinogenic.

Increase Intake of Foods Rich in Beta Carotene and Vitamin C in the Daily Diet   Carrots, spinach, apricots, peaches and tomatoes are all rich in beta carotene, a precursor of active vitamin A, which has been associated with a decreased risk of cancers of the larynx, oesophagus and lung. Vitamin C can inhibit the formation of nitrosamines and may therefore be able to decrease the risk of cancer.

Vitamin A and Cancer

A diet that contains adequate amounts of foods rich in vitamin A such as dark green leafy vegetables, carrots and apricots has been found to reduce the risk of cancers. These dark green or orange vegetables and fruits contain beta carotene, the plant pigment which is converted to vitamin A in the body.

The connection between vitamin A and cancer was first made as early as 1920. Since then vitamin A and its related compounds have been studied extensively with regard to their effect on the development of cancer. Until recently the main thrust of research was aimed at finding how vitamin A works in cancer prevention, but the interest has now shifted to beta carotene. This is because there is a strong correlation between a high intake of foods containing beta carotene and lower risks of cancers of the lung and stomach. Numerous studies have compared the incidence of various types of cancer with vitamin A or beta carotene intake, one of the largest of which involved monitoring the diets of nearly 250,000 people in Japan over a ten-year period. The findings from this study showed that the daily consumption of vegetables with high levels of beta carotene reduced the risk of lung, colon, stomach, prostate and cervical cancer.

Vitamin C and Cancer

Vitamin C is another anticancer vitamin. Firstly, people who consume vitamin C-rich foods, such as citrus fruits, have a reduced risk of stomach and throat cancers; and secondly, vitamin C inactivates the cancer-causing nitrosamines. In the absence of vitamin C, the nitrates (which are found in cigarettes, smoked meat and processed foods) are converted into nitrosamines. The presence of vitamin C blocks the formation of these nitrosamines thus reducing the risk of cancer developing.

Vitamin E and Selenium, and Cancer

There is increasing evidence that selenium levels in the body decline as cancer progresses. Some experts believe that selenium exerts its protective role by virtue of its function as a cofactor for certain enzyme systems responsible for the metabolism of fat.

Research shows that selenium and vitamin E are two powerful antioxidant nutrients that act together in the prevention and growth of cancer. They prevent cell damage by the highly reactive free radicals. There is increasing evidence that people living in an area where the selenium content of the soil is poor have high rates of cancer of the lymph system, the digestive tract, lungs and breast. Additionally, vitamin E protects fats in the body from free radical damage.

Erroneously called a disease of the twentieth century, cancer is not in fact a new disease. It is the high incidence of the disease that has made it appear so. This is due to our modern lifestyle and depleted diet.

HEART DISEASE

Coronary heart disease is the commonest cause of death in the UK, and the second commonest cause of death in women. One in three of the male population in the UK will eventually suffer from coronary heart disease, and one in five will die of a heart attack. The total number of deaths from heart attacks is estimated to be between 500,000 and 800,000. In the USA, which has one of the highest incidences of heart disease in the world, more than a million people a year suffer heart attacks and fifty per cent of them die as a result. These frightening statistics are repeated throughout Europe, Canada, Australia and other so-called 'developed countries'. The disease is also on the increase in the Third World.

What Really is a Heart Attack?

The heart is a pump that sends the blood through the body. To start the cycle the blood first passes through the lungs to pick up the oxygen that we have breathed in. This oxygenated blood is carried round the body in tubes called arteries, and returned to the heart through tubes called veins.

A heart attack occurs when a clot of blood blocks one of the main arteries – the coronary artery (in Latin *corona* means 'a crown') – or one of its main branches. When the walls of the artery are blocked by a fatty porridge-like substance made of fat, cholesterol and a protein called atheroma, blood flow is restricted. When the artery, already narrowed by atheroma deposits, is suddenly filled with a blood clot, a heart attack occurs.

There are a number of risk factors that precipitate a heart attack:

- *Smoking*: worsens atheroma and also promotes the blood clot.
- *Excessive fat in the bloodstream.*
- *Stress*: makes the blood thicker and promotes a higher viscosity in the blood flow.
- *Raised blood pressure.*
- *Increase in the stickiness of the platelets in our blood*: platelets are

47

small sticky bodies that circulate along with red and white blood cells and stick together like little blobs of glue becoming the basis of clot formation.

When the partially blocked artery is completely blocked, the heart is deprived of its blood supply. This registers as an acute pain. In the process part of the heart muscle may actually die and the heart is damaged. The damaged heart can no longer function correctly and in some cases will fail, resulting in death.

What is Cholesterol?

A word that invariably accompanies any discussion on heart attack is 'cholesterol'. Blacklisted as a dietary component, it is one of the most misunderstood and maligned substances in human nutrition. There is a body of opinion that believes that lowering cholesterol in the diet will greatly reduce the risk of heart attack, while there are others who insist it would not make an iota of difference. It is neither within the scope nor the intention of this book to delve into the academics of this debate, but the subject requires some elaboration.

It is now firmly established that excessive fat in the diet results in high blood cholesterol levels and that, in turn, these increase the risk of a heart attack. This is because cholesterol becomes deposited in the walls of the arteries, causing a roughening of the inner lining of the blood vessels (atherosclerosis). In atherosclerosis, blood platelets tend to collect, forming a clot around damaged areas, thus narrowing the artery. As stated before, these clots can eventually block the blood supply, causing a heart attack.

The Vital Role of Cholesterol

Because cholesterol is blacklisted, its necessity in the body is often not appreciated. In fact every cell in the body contains cholesterol. This fatty substance resides in our cell walls, where it helps to maintain the rigid structure of the cells. A properly intact cell wall is necessary to protect delicate cell contents and so cholesterol's structural role is vital. Cholesterol is also needed for the formation of bile salts and is vital in the body for the production of steroid hormones. It is the raw material from which the sex and adrenal hormones are made. However, we do not need to obtain cholesterol from our food because the body is able to produce its own supplies. So, cholesterol is not a new substance that has afflicted us only in this century. What has happened is that we have got the balance wrong.

Cholesterol is manufactured in the liver. In order to transport cholesterol through the body, the body produces droplets made of fat and protein called LDLs and HDLs. The main particle involved in ferrying cholesterol is called LDL (low density lipoprotein). The LDL takes the cholesterol from the liver and transports it to the parts of the body that need it.

Increasingly now, the carrier system for cholesterol, as well as the total blood cholesterol, is considered important. The HDLs (high density lipoproteins) carry cholesterol to the liver, thereby effectively removing or 'scavenging' it from the body. On the other hand, LDLs transport cholesterol to tissues where it is deposited. Problems arise when there is an excess of LDL cholesterol and it is dumped in areas where it should not be. One of these areas is the coronary artery.

Diet to Reduce Cholesterol Levels

Anything which increases HDL and reduces LDL in the blood is likely to be effective in reducing the risk of heart disease. According to recent clinical trials, garlic appears to be one such substance (more on this in Chapter 6). In a recently published study, an odourless aged garlic preparation (see p. 83) was found to lower total blood cholesterol, increase HDL and lower LDL.

Lecithin supplementation also appears to be effective in reducing blood cholesterol. Lecithin is a natural emulsifier (that is, it can bring about the mixing of fats and water-based fluids – two normally incompatible substances). This means that lecithin can solubilize and mobilize cholesterol deposits which can help prevent or reverse atherosclerosis.

Other supplements that have been found beneficial in reducing blood cholesterol levels include niacin and high vitamin C intake. This is probably because vitamin C is needed for the transformation of cholesterol to bile salts. Efficient bile salt production means excess cholesterol is rarely available to build up and cause harm.

Fish oils from fatty fish such as salmon have been found to have extensive benefits in cardiovascular conditions, not least at lowering LDL blood cholesterol, with a simultaneous entrainment of HDL.

Vitamin Guide

Fish oil is the oil which is squeezed from the muscle of oily fish. This is different from cod liver oil which is squeezed from the liver and not the flesh. Cod liver oil is rich in vitamins A and D but does not necessarily have as much essential fatty acid content as fish oil.

The vital ingredients in fish oil are two tongue-twisting fatty acids – eicosapentaenoic acid and docosahexaenoic acid – EPA and DHA for short. These essential fatty acids called 'omega-3', which are obtained by the fish from plankton, are required by both fish and humans. However, neither humans nor fish can manufacture these themselves and rely on obtaining them from food. (See Chapter 6 on fish oils.)

How Much is Too Much?

The answer to this question has to take into account the fact that our bodies do not actually need a dietary source of cholesterol at all. The liver makes its own supply of cholesterol and, quite simply, can make enough without an additional external source being necessary.

Estimates suggest that, to minimize health risks, the amount of cholesterol in the diet should be no more than 200–300mg per day. This is only a small allowance – the equivalent of one egg.

Some Cholesterol Rich Foods

	Cholesterol mg/100g.
Brains	2,000
Egg yolk	1,480
Kidney	804
Whole egg	504
Liver	438
Heart (beef)	274
Lobster	180
Shrimps	150
Double cream	133

Blood Triglycerides

Triglycerides are a lesser known substance also responsible for an elevated risk of heart disease. Some experts believe that triglycerides are even more important indicators of risk than cholesterol.

A high level of triglycerides can increase the risk of death from heart disease, since it renders the blood more likely to produce clots, makes the blood more viscous and therefore less able to squeeze through narrow blood vessels.

Once again the omega-3 polyunsaturates from fish oils can dramatically lower triglyceride levels (by as much as thirty per cent), and therefore reduce risk of heart attack.

The Fibre Connection in Heart Disease

The fibre in food has an active effect against cholesterol. This is because fibre tends to bind with cholesterol in the gut and so prevent its absorption in the body. Another advantage is that fibre also encourages the growth of intestinal bacteria, some of which degrade the cholesterol into products which are very poorly absorbed.

Plant foods also contain another component which is, quite literally, nature's 'cholesterol neutralizer'. The substance is beta-sitosterol and can be regarded as the plant equivalent of cholesterol. However, far from having the same harmful effects as cholesterol, beta-sitosterol actually blocks the absorption of cholesterol in the intestine. It does this by competing with cholesterol for the same absorption sites on the intestinal wall. The body 'mistakes' beta-sitosterol for cholesterol, tries to absorb it, finds that it cannot and therefore releases the beta-sitosterol again. Meanwhile the cholesterol has passed through the body unabsorbed. Unfortunately, modern oil seed processing techniques remove much of this valuable substance from the final product.

It is important to emphasize that, while most of the blood cholesterol-lowering substances such as garlic, fish oils, vitamin C, niacin, and lecithin, achieve their purpose by mobilizing cholesterol so that it can be transported to the liver, beta-sitosterol is a notable exception. By virtue of the fact that cholesterol is converted in the liver to bile salts, much cholesterol actually ends up back in the intestine again, where there is a danger that it will simply be reabsorbed. Therefore, although garlic, lecithin, and fish oils do have a well-documented value in reducing cholesterol levels, their efficiency is even further enhanced by the simultaneous presence of beta-sitosterol in the diet. An example of an ideal combination is lecithin and beta-sitosterol. The former mobilizes cholesterol from the deposition sites while the latter ensures that the cholesterol is not reabsorbed back into the body. It also blocks off any 'fresh' dietary cholesterol.

Cholesterol alone does not cause heart attacks, but an elevated blood cholesterol is invariably present in a potential heart victim. By taking care to lower blood cholesterol, untold suffering can avoided.

STRESS

We all experience stress – in fact a certain amount of stress is good for us as it keeps us motivated. But there are times when stress appears to take over our lives and it is then that it can affect our health. Its effects have been extensively researched. Depression, chronic anxiety and its weakening effect upon the human system have all been attributed to stress.

The dictionary definition of stress is 'a mentally or emotionally disruptive or disquieting influence'. Bereavement, divorce, relationship problems, financial difficulties, redundancies are all familiar examples of emotionally disruptive influences.

There are all sorts of reasons why people suffer from stress. One of them is change. A common link between all the possible causes is our deep-seated anxiety about change. We are all vulnerable to change and as we go through life most of us learn to adapt successfully to it, but at times it can be especially difficult to cope with. As we go through life, a continual bombardment by the problems of daily living, albeit trivial, can disrupt mental and emotional equilibrium in the same way as a major calamity.

While mental stress affects our health, specific mention of physical conditions must also be made to complete the picture. Smoking (both active and passive), poor ventilation, very high or low temperatures, atmospheric pollution, in conjunction with bad dietary habits and poor nutrition all take their toll on the human body.

Much of the research into stress has involved observation of the sympathetic nervous system. This is one of the two divisions of the autonomic nervous system, responsible for regulating unconscious body functions. This system comprises sympathetic nerves and ganglia (nervous relay stations). Sympathetic nerves act by releasing substances called adrenaline and noradrenaline. These tend to quicken the heart rate, raise the blood pressure, release glucose, and slow the digestive processes. The large quantities of adrenaline circulate throughout the body thus preparing the body for emergency action. This adrenaline released by the body has been generally termed the 'fight or flight' response. It prepares the body to cope with sudden physical emergencies such as accidents or any harmful events that the brain perceives. This 'fight or flight' response is also stimulated by stress factors.

The body is able to cope with occasional stress at a certain level. However, if it keeps recurring there is a danger of physical and psychological effects on the body. When one is faced with a situation of prolonged stress the seemingly trivial, everyday problems become unmanageable. Anxiety sets in. One may feel tense and at times hyperactive. What is sometimes not known is that the long-term damage can be serious. Strokes, insomnia, ulcers, headaches, high blood pressure, high blood cholesterol levels can all be induced by prolonged stress. It also affects the digestive process, encouraging ulcer formation and gastric upsets. Stress is also known to affect the immune system, diminishing our ability to fight disease (see chapter 2).

Whenever possible, practical measures such as discussing your problems with a doctor, partner or a counsellor should be taken; and harmful habits such as smoking and alcohol consumption should be tackled. Exercise will improve circulation, control body weight and blood pressure, and will also provide an outlet for mental tension resulting in relaxation – which is mandatory for good health.

In addition, stress increases the body's requirements of nearly all nutrients. When we are under stress, good nutrition becomes even more important because stress draws on our natural resources causing the body to function less efficiently. It should be said that in addition to dietary measures and taking certain antistress supplements, exercise and general changes in lifestyle can be effective means of combating stress.

Antistress Nutrients

- The B vitamins play an important role in helping us resist the effects of stress. As they are not stored for any length of time in the body, they are the first of the nutrients to develop deficiencies.
- Vitamin C with bioflavonoids.
- Vitamin E helps to relieve stress-induced fatigue and enables the brain cells to obtain adequate supplies of oxygen.

- Calcium offers protection against osteoporosis. Taken at bedtime it aids natural healthy sleep.
- Magnesium guards against depression. It is necessary for calcium metabolism and is depleted by stress. Alcohol increases the body's requirement of the mineral.
- Zinc helps counteract depression and increases mental alertness.

5

Nutritional Therapy

The doctor has only one task: to heal the sick . . . it is of no consequence which means he uses. Hippocrates (460–370 BC)

THE STUDY OF NUTRITION has come a long way in the last hundred years. The link between food and deficiency diseases has gone beyond the notion of prevention and treatment of disease. Research is now uncovering the link between diet and behaviour, intelligence and mental health – for example, the emotional changes that sometimes precede menstruation partially result from nutrient imbalances (see Chapter 3).

The whole science of nutrition has passed through various phases. The first phase was nutrition in the *treatment* of disease. Scurvy and pellagra, which claimed thousands of lives, were eliminated by the simple treatment of providing the missing nutrients from the diet. The concept of a well-balanced diet gained currency; and the definition of a well-balanced diet was one that prevented the onset of disease.

The second phase of development was, nutrition for the *prevention* of disease. Research showed that there was a strong relationship between the dietary intake of nutrients and the development, progression and cure of diseases other than deficiency diseases. Soon the link between nutrition and infectious diseases, as well as diseases of the heart and bone was established. Further research uncovered the impact of nutrition on immunity, the prevention of cancer and other degenerative diseases, the so called 'diseases of civilization'.

Now the latest nutritional thinking is focused on the additional roles of nutrition in stress, moods, the ageing process and even intellectual development. The science of nutrition has widened to include the fields of psychology, and research is constantly uncovering new links between diet and behaviour, mental health and intelligence. The complexities of the issues raise fundamental questions on the concept of a well-balanced diet, and beg the redefinition of a diet that provides optimal (and not just adequate) levels of nutrients.

In understanding the role of diet and disease, it must be understood that nutritional therapy does not offer magic pills or potions to cure or prevent specific ailments. The first and foremost consideration is to enjoy a diet that is low in fats, high in fibre, and which has adequate levels of vitamins and minerals. Additionally, a good diet should contain a variety of fresh fruit and vegetables, whole grain breads, cereals, beans and pulses, and small amounts of lean meat, chicken and fish.

Where there is a deficiency of certain nutrients, or the body is depleted of various nutrients, supplements in the form of pills, capsules or liquids may be taken in consultation with a qualified nutritionist or a dietary therapist. This will ensure that the correct balances between nutrients are maintained.

Vitamins and minerals are a collection of interrelated substances and the body uses them synergistically. For example both vitamin D and magnesium are necessary for the proper utilization of calcium. Vitamin C is necessary for iron absorption, and vitamin E protects vitamins A and D from oxidation.

On the other hand, some nutrients taken on their own deplete others. For example, zinc taken in large quantities can cause a depletion of copper and can exacerbate ailments. Therefore the haphazard taking of supplements can be wasteful, inefficient and may even cause deficiency of other nutrients, thus creating an imbalance in the system. (For information regarding correct supplementation, see Part Two.)

Drugs produce dietary deficiences by either destroying nutrients or using them up. It is regrettable that the majority of the medical profession take the attitude that a prescribed drug is the total cure for an ailment. A nutritional councillor will look at drug interactions and nutritional deficiencies on a carefully balanced supplements programme.

In this chapter we shall look at some common conditions where nutritional therapy can be an effective alternative to drug therapy.

ALZHEIMER'S DISEASE

What Is It?
It is a slow, progressive and irreversible loss of memory.

What Causes It?
The nerves that originate in the middle region of the brain and extend into the cortex become tangled with abnormal protein deposits. As this condition progresses, the blood vessels supplying oxygen and nutrients to these cells degenerate and the cells die. The concentrations of chemical messengers between these nerve cells (called neurotransmitters) decline, resulting in memory loss. As the damage spreads, long-term memory is progressively affected as are other body functions such as bladder control, co-ordination and many others.

Dietary Factors
While it is not known whether abnormal levels of aluminium are the cause or effect of Alzheimer's disease, excessive accumulation of aluminium is associated with nervous system disorders. Aluminium cookware, certain medications, and sundries such as antacid and antiperspirant deodorants, all contain aluminium. A sufficient intake of calcium and zinc is known to reduce aluminium absorption.

Choline   Lecithin is the common name for a dietary substance called phosphatidycholine which is the best source of choline. It is also a constituent of acetycholine, the neurotransmitter that is depleted in Alzheimer's disease. Intake of choline or lecithin can be useful in the early stages of short-term memory loss.

Vitamins   Several vitamin deficiencies have been linked to Alzheimer's disease – for instance, a long-term B12 deficiency. It has been found that over seventy per cent of older persons who are deficient in vitamin B12 also suffer from the disease. Patients with dementia also show long-term poor intake of vitamin C and folic acid – two nutrients essential for cell maintance and normal division.

Until more definitive evidence is available, a diet low in aluminium, fat and sugar, and high in zinc, B vitamins and choline is recommended.

ARTHRITIS

What Is It?
Arthritis is inflammation of the joints, the two most common types being rheumatoid arthritis and osteoarthritis. Rheumatoid arthritis is the inflammation of the lining of the joints. Although any joints

can be affected, the small joints of the hands and feet are the most susceptible. Osteoarthritis is the degeneration of the cartilage in the joints. The most likely parts to be affected are the joints in the feet, and the joints of the weight-bearing bones.

What Causes It?
Osteoarthritis is the most common type of arthritis and is caused by prolonged physical stress and injury. Symptoms include stiffness, soreness and pain.

Rheumatoid arthritis is probably due to the malfunction of the immune defence system, and is therefore known as an auto-immune disease. It is a result of the immune system producing antibodies against its own healthy organs and tissues, instead of against invading bacteria and viruses.

Symptoms typically fluctuate, with periods of remission following weeks or months of disability. Symptoms include swelling (caused by accumulation of fluids in the linings of the joints), stiffness and pain.

Dietary Factors
Nutrient Deficiency   Poor dietary intake of some nutrients is associated with rheumatoid arthritis. What is not known is whether poor nutrition causes arthritis or is a result of the disease. Arthritis patients are commonly deficient in vitamin D, folic acid, vitamin B6, vitamin C, zinc and iron.

Antioxidants   Increased intake of antioxidant nutrients such as vitamin E and selenium reduce free radical damage to joint linings. It is this damage that results in the accumulation of fluids, swelling and consequent pain in rheumatoid arthritis patients.

Fish Oils   Rheumatoid arthritis patients report improvements in morning stiffness when they take fish oil capsules. Folk medicine in many countries recommends 'oiling creaking joints' with fish oil. The idea that fish oils somehow help 'lubricate' joints like rusty door hinges is fallacious: the error lies in the simplistic explanation of the effect rather than the effect itself!

Clinical tests have shown that fish oil extracts treat arthritis effectively. A product combining fish oils with evening primrose oil used in a large trial, organized by orthopaedic specialists and involving hundreds of rheumatoid arthritis sufferers, was found to be sufficiently effective to allow a large number of patients to reduce the doses of their anti-arthritic drugs – a vivid illustration of partial replacement of conventional medicine with a natural substance free from side effects! (For further explanation on fish oils see Chapter 6.)

The fatty acids in fish oils known as eicosapentaenoic acid (EPA) and the linoleic acid found in plant oils which is an essential fatty acid can be converted by our cells into anti-inflammatory substances easing the joint pain and stiffness.

All in all, good nutrition improves some symptoms and in many cases counteracts the side effects of medication. An adequate intake of calcium and vitamin D helps prevent bone loss associated with the use of steroids in the treatment of rheumatoid arthritis. Symptoms of osteoarthritis diminish if a healthy diet is followed, and can also often be helped by weight reduction.

THE COMMON COLD

The common cold is the most widespread infectious health complaint and is caused by virus infection. The virus first attacks the nose and throat and later spreads to the respiratory tubes. Chances of infection are heightened by stress, exhaustion and chronic sickness.

Dietary Factors
All the nutrients that assist in maintaining a healthy immune system are important. Cold viruses change constantly, so immunity acquired from one infection will not necessarily protect one from further attacks – all the more reason for maintaining a healthy immune system.

Vitamin C   Vitamin C is popularly known to have a positive effect in preventing the common cold. It stimulates the immune system by increasing the production and activity of specialized white blood cells. Vitamin C deficiency is related to an increased susceptibility to infection and a reduction in white blood cell formation (white blood cells carry the body's fighting forces).

Zinc   Because certain viruses cannot survive in a zinc-rich environment, zinc supplementation has a direct effect on viral growth and hence on the common cold. Zinc also stimulates the immune system. This mineral affects the production and activity of T-cells (see Chapter 2) in the immune system.

Low blood levels of zinc are associated with reduced resistance to infections due to an impaired immune function, while optimal intake of zinc will protect the body from infections. However, care must be exercised to limit zinc intake to 20mg per day (RDA 12–15 mg/day). Higher doses may result in a secondary deficiency of copper, as zinc may interfere with copper absorption.

OSTEOPOROSIS

What Is It?
'Thinning of the bones' – a disease whereby the skeleton loses its mass and becomes fragile so that fractures can occur very easily. A post-menopausal woman may have only fifty per cent of her original bone mass if osteoporosis develops, a man only twenty-five per cent. Osteoporosis is ten times more likely in women than in men.

What Causes It?
Lack of sufficient calcium during life to build up a solid bone mass, and/or falling oestrogen levels in the menopause, particularly if inadequate attention has been paid to diet and nutrition.

Dietary Factors
Vitamin D and Phytic Acid Calcium must be taken regularly throughout life. Levels of calcium during the first thirty-five years will have a bearing on the likelihood of the later development of osteoporosis (see page 35). Calcium requires other nutrients in order to be absorbed by the body, notably magnesium and vitamin D. Vitamin D is converted into a hormone which encourages calcium retention in the bones. Phytic acid, present in cereal foods, also hinders absorption of calcium. For those with a tendency to kidney stones, calcium should be taken in conjunction with magnesium and vitamin B6.

ECZEMA AND PSORIASIS

What Are They?
Eczema is a skin complaint characterized by inflammation, irritation, and the shedding of dry scales. Infection can develop which then leads to further inflammation, severe soreness and pus-filled spots and scabs. Psoriasis is very similar to eczema in that it is also

a skin complaint consisting of skin lesions which may be dry and scaly or pus-filled and scaly. The lining of the skin's blood vessels and the skin cells are abnormal, as is the rate of production of new skin.

What Causes Them?
Eczema exists in three forms: endogenous, atopic and seborrhoeic. The first is caused by reactions within the body itself; the second by external causes, usually an allergic reaction or an irritant which has come into contact with the skin; and the third type, seborrhoeic, is common amongst teenage boys, and men in their early twenties and is a result of excessive production of sebum (skin lubricant).

   Psoriasis is not caused by any one particular factor; but stress, injury, infection and drugs (beta blockers, non-steroidal anti-inflammatory drugs, and lithium) are common catalysts.

Dietary Factors
A wholefood diet is the key to eliminating endogenous eczema.

Milk allergy   Cow's milk may have to be replaced with a soya or casein-based product. In the case of atopic eczema, discovery of the irritant and its exclusion will remedy the complaint.

Fasting   For both eczema and psoriasis some practitioners recommend a fast in which only water, herbal teas and fruit and vegetable juices are allowed. At the end of the cure a wholefood diet is prescribed.

General Supplementation   The following supplements may be helpful in treating both these conditions:

- A multivitamin/mineral complex.
- Vitamin A.
- Vitamin E.
- Chelated zinc.
- Propolis.
- Rosehip vitamin C with bioflavonoids.
- Fish oil capsules.
- Evening primrose oil.

HAYFEVER

What Is It?
A seasonal complaint arising in summer, consisting of a blocked nose, running, itchy eyes and nose, violent sneezing, a dry cough, and sometimes even asthmatic attacks.

What Causes It?
An allergic reaction to pollen. Histamine (produced by the body)
causes inflammation of the mucous membranes lining the nose, eyes,
and air passages.

Dietary Factors
Anti-histamines are commonly prescribed to relieve inflammation.
However, side effects include drowsiness, lack of co-ordination,
chest tightness, blurred vision and tingling hands, and only fifty
per cent of users derive any benefit from anti-histamines.

General Supplementation   Vitamin C with bioflavonoids has an anti-
histamine effect at dosages of 200–500mg daily. Vitamin B5, usually
taken in conjunction with vitamin E, also has an anti-histamine
effect. In addition, vitamins A and the B-complex, magnesium,
calcium, potassium, selenium and zinc all help hayfever, so the
best bet may be to take a good multivitamin/mineral supplement.
    Relief can also be acquired by following a diet high in fresh
fruit and vegetables, and a combination of high protein and high
carbohydrates but excluding most dairy products.

MULTIPLE SCLEROSIS

What Is It?
Multiple sclerosis is a disease which attacks the white matter of the
central nervous system (CNS). This white matter, called myelin,
forms protective, insulating sheaths around the nerve cells found
inside the brain and in the outer layers of the spinal cord. These
nerves are part of the body's telegraph wires connecting the brain
with the sensory organs and muscles. Myelin is destroyed at one or
more sites (hence the adjective 'multiple'), and then scar tissue is
built up by the body in an attempt to repair the damage.

What Causes It?
Unfortunately, despite ongoing research, the cause of multiple
sclerosis has not yet been definitively identified. However, infection, auto-immunity, and possibly food allergy, as well as a shortage
of essential fatty acids (EFAs), are believed to contribute to
multiple sclerosis.

Dietary Factors
Evening Primrose Oil Because a shortage of EFAs is common amongst multiple sclerosis sufferers, evening primrose oil is often recommended. Evening primrose oil can bring about significant relief, especially during the early stages. Further, myelin is rich in EFAs, and therefore a defective EFA metabolism may make myelin vulnerable to attack. Additionally, multiple sclerosis has a higher incidence amongst people whose intake of saturated fats is high, while that of polyunsaturated fats (PUFAs include EFAs) is low.

General Supplementation A multivitamin/mineral complex, vitamin B-complex, vitamin C with bioflavonoids, vitamin E, and zinc are likely to promote general good health and strengthen the immune system and therefore be of some benefit where multiple sclerosis has occurred. Vitamin B12 supplements may also be helpful as multiple sclerosis patients are often deficient in this vitamin.

CANDIDA ALBICANS – THE YEAST SYNDROME

What Is It?
Candida infects the skin, mouth and vagina. The yeast syndrome affects other parts of the body causing cystitis, skin rashes, overall loss of vitality, muscular weakness, and long bouts of fatigue.

What Causes It?
The natural yeast fungus overgrows and causes problems. A prolonged course of antibiotics or steroids, poor diet, chronic stress, environmental pollution, ageing, cancer, AIDS or TB are all causes of candida and the yeast syndrome.

Dietary Factors
The objectives are to reduce the yeast growth, and boost the immune system which, if it had been in good working order in the first place, would have protected the body from yeast syndrome.

Elimination of Yeast Products This is essential. Mushrooms and other edible fungi, bread, sugar, honey, blue cheese, alcohol, vinegar and pickled foods (anything fermented), should be excluded.

A Wholefood Diet A balanced, wholefood diet is the key factor for a return to health. This means: fish, offal, eggs, poultry and vegetarian dishes to supply protein; fresh vegetables to supply fibre, vitamins and minerals (fruit must be avoided because of its sugar content – at least for the first six weeks); cereals, grains, pulses and nuts to supply fibre and complex carbohydrates; plant and seed oils and their products as substitutes for butter and other high-fat dairy foods.

Supplementation against the Yeast Syndrome   A high potency vitamin B-complex is helpful to ease stress and maximize the energy from carbohydrate foods. Vitamin C with bioflavonoids speeds the healing process, strengthens the immune system and combats stress. Biotin is thought to have a direct effect on controlling candidal growth and combats chronic fatigue. Zinc increases mental alertness and has a powerful antioxidant action. Garlic is widely recommended for candida because it seems to mop up the toxins produced by the yeast. It also kills yeast itself and stimulates the immune system. *Lactobacillus acidophilus* is useful since it is a friendly intestinal bacterium which normally helps keep candida growth within safe limits but which is destroyed by antibiotics.

ANTIBIOTICS

Seeing this heading under a chapter entitled Nutritional Therapy has very likely made you do a double-take. However, it is actually not out of place since the 'broad-spectrum' antibiotics (i.e. a combination of antibiotics) if taken for too long will kill bacteria. This means that even the friendly bacteria which the body needs are destroyed – so whilst one health problem may be cured by antibiotics, another is often generated.

Candida (see above) may well come about after a prolonged course of antibiotics, and a course of *Lactobacillus acidophilus* should follow immediately after any course of antibiotics to help repopulate the gut with friendly bacteria. Diarrhoea can also result after antibiotics because the intestinal lining is irritated and inflamed. If diarrhoea occurs during the use of antibiotics you should inform your doctor as alternative medication may be available. Diarrhoea itself interferes with the body's fluid balance, depletes the body of its store of nutrients, and can lead to muscular weakness, lethargy and fatigue. Potassium supplements will help, as will apples, peaches and bananas all of which are rich in potassium.

Skin rashes are another side effect of antibiotic use, and this is the reaction of an overtaxed immune system. Nutrients which strengthen the immune system are therefore useful: vitamin C with bioflavonoids, zinc, evening primrose oil, vitamin B-complex and a good multivitamin.

PROBIOTICS

The opposite to antibiotics? In many ways, yes. After friendly and unfriendly bacteria have been destroyed by a course of antibiotics, the body starts to repopulate its bacteria supply. Hopefully the correct balance of friendly and non-friendly bacteria is re-established, but there is every likelihood that the unfriendly bacteria will overrun the friendly – resulting in candida, flatulence and a painful stomach. Supplementation with probiotics, the friendly bacteria, is now a common measure is promoting health.

As I said earlier, a course of *Lactobacillus acidophilus* is advisable after antibiotics. Bifidobacteria are also friendly. Some UK supermarkets now sell 'live' natural and fruited yogurts which contain the live bacteria *Lactobacillus acidophilus* and Bifidobacteria, but care should be taken to choose a quality brand since some so-called 'live' yogurts are about as lively as a cemetery.

PRE-OP/POST-OP CARE

Jokes about the quality of hospital food are rather poignant. There you have a building full of sick people who have undergone surgery, some of which is major but all of which is a shock to the system. Just when the body needs all the help it can get to recover from the stress it has undergone, the patient often turns away from the hospital food because it is unappetizing or poorly cooked.

If you or a member of your family is due to undergo surgery, give your body a helping hand to recovery by boosting your immune system before you go into hospital. Vitamin E, selenium, GLA, zinc citrate, vitamin C with bioflavonoids, vitamin A, vitamin B-complex all boost the immune system. Once you come out of hospital, continue taking at least a general supplement, and follow a healthy diet.

6

Wonder Supplements – Myth or Magic?

Let nature work freely in everything
Jean Jacques Rousseau (1712–1778)

A MATTER OF FAT

FATS *PER SE* ARE not all bad news. Some are good, some bad, some necessary, and some necessary to avoid! Until very recently the clear message from nutritionists was that butter is bad for you and that polyunsaturates are good for you. Now we know that the matter is not that simple. Lately we have been subjected to much conflicting advice on which fats are good for us and which are bad. Basically there are two types of fats: storage and structural.

Storage fats are predominantly saturated fats – the commonest type being derived from animal fats. These provide a long term supply of energy to the body in times of food or energy shortage. *Structural fats* are mainly composed of polyunsaturated fats and are found in plants, vegetables and some fish. They are vital for our metabolic processes as required for the functioning of certain enzymes.

Dietary Intake of Fats

On average our diet provides between forty and sixty per cent of our daily energy intake as fats. It is clear from diet surveys that we consume far too much cholesterol and saturated fats, most of which is unnecessary because our bodies can and do synthesize cholesterol from other sources.

On the other hand, the essential fats required by the body to build structural fats cannot be made by the body, and hence their presence in the diet is of the utmost importance. Unfortunately, it is these essential fats that are either completely lacking or are not present in sufficient amounts in our food. Modern eating habits, food processing and intensive animal rearing practices ensure that our diet is severely deficient in these essential fats.

Growth failure, dry skin, increased water loss and a number of metabolic disorders are the results of a deficiency of these polyunsaturated fats. As these nutrients for body growth and function have to be provided in the diet, they are called essential fatty acids.

Essential Fatty Acids

There are two families of EFAs (namely Omega-3 and Omega-6) the parent members of which can both be found in vegetable oils. However, further conversion into more useful acid derivatives such as gamma linolenic acid (GLA) and eicosapentaenoic acids (EPA) is severely limited by factors such as age, diet and hormonal condition. That is why fish oils and evening primrose oil, providing a direct source of EPA and GLA respectively, can be so beneficial. Diets high in saturated fats, cholesterol and trans fatty acids reduce the body's ability to produce these polyunsaturated fatty acids.

Two Major Functions of EFAs

1. *Converting Nutrients into Energy*   All cell membranes contain fats which are important in maintaining the integrity of the membrane and providing sites for many physiological processes to take place. To put it simply, if there is a deficiency of EFAs, the process in which nutrients are converted into body energy becomes inefficient. This lack of energy leads to poor growth and an impairment of body function.

2. *Precursors of Prostaglandins*   Prostaglandins are hormone-like substances. It has now been established that these prostaglandins are produced from EFAs. They also help regulate blood pressure, stimulate the immune system and maintain good cardiovascular function.

The Role of EFAs in Disease Management
Dietary deficiency of EFAs results in altered membrane function, dermatosis, weight loss and eczema.

Individual fatty acids have been successfully used in the management of a number of ailments. For example, supplementation with gamma linolenic acid (GLA) has resulted in successful treatment of eczema, PMT, hypercholesterolaemia and cardiovascular disorders. It is interesting to note that these conditions are largely attributed to metabolic disorders resulting from our bad eating habits and our Western lifestyle.

Supplementing with eicosapentaenoic acid (EPA) has been proven to help reduce blood triglyceride levels and has inhibited blood clotting in patients with heart problems. Numerous studies are currently underway to evaluate the role of some of the individual polyunsaturated fatty acids in managing immune system-related disorders.

THE EVENING PRIMROSE OIL STORY

First brought to Europe from Virginia in the 1600s, the evening primrose plant quickly became a garden favourite. At the same time herbalists began to recognize its health properties. Today, there is extensive research that supports the many claims in which evening primrose oil is so clearly beneficial.

So what is it about this unassuming yellow flower that is now known to possess such remarkable health giving properties? The simple answer is its gamma linolenic acid (GLA) content.

The key to the plant's nutritional secret is the oil that is collected from its seeds. Most vegetable oils contain linoleic acid – an essential fatty acid – and the normal diet is quite sufficient in this. However, before this essential fatty acid can be used by the body, it has to be converted into prostaglandin E1, and unfortunately this conversion is fraught with difficulties and can easily be blocked. Viruses, cholesterol, saturated fatty acids, alcohol, insufficient insulin, radiation, vitamin and mineral deficiency, and the ageing process all contribute to blocking or adversely affecting this conversion.

As evening primrose oil has an unusually high amount of GLA, it can potentially avoid all these blockages. Such a source of dietary GLA can therefore be extremely valuable since it can skip these potential blockages and provide the material from which prostaglandin E1 can easily be produced.

Conversion from LA to GLA is blocked by:

Saturated fats (butter, dairy produce),
alcohol, aging, viruses,
Alpha Linolenic Acid (blackcurrant oil, linseed oil),
excess sugar, tartrazine.

Conversion of GLA is blocked by:-
steroids, Alpha Linolenic Acid

Linoleic Acid
↓
requires Zinc & Magnesium, B6, Biotin
↓
Gamma Linolenic Acid
↓
requires B6, Calcium, Zinc
↓
Dihomo Gamma Linolenic Acid
↓
requires Niacin, Vitamin C, Zinc, Selenium
↓
Prostaglandin E1

Further, if the body cannot make sufficient GLA and does not receive a dietary supply then some of the body systems can be impaired. Evening primrose oil can help in conditions such as PMT, eczema, rheumatoid arthritis and cholesterol control. This list is by no means exhaustive, and new research is now suggesting that ME (myalgic encephalomyelitis, also known as chronic fatigue syndrome) sufferers may also benefit, as may hyperactive children and alcoholics.

Premenstrual Tension
One of the biggest benefits of evening primrose oil is to women who suffer from premenstrual tension. Specific prostaglandins are needed to help regulate the hormonal control of the menstrual cycle. Sufficient GLA to form the prostaglandins can be immensely helpful. Trials suggest that four to eight 500mg capsules taken daily in the second two weeks of the cycle can dramatically ease symptoms such as breast tenderness, irritability, anxiety, swollen abdomen, and so on. However, women may need to take evening primrose oil for up to five complete cycles before the full benefits are noted (see Chapter 3).

Eczema

Both adults and children can benefit from using evening primrose oil for eczema. Eczema is thought to be specifically associated with a deficiency of the enzyme needed to form GLA from linoleic acid – so a direct supply of GLA can be very useful. Research suggests that a minimum of four 500mg capsules daily in adults, and two a day in children, is needed to improve itching, but eight to twelve 500mg capsules a day in adults, and four a day in children is probably required to improve the overall severity of the disease.

Cholesterol/High Blood Pressure

Fish oils have received more publicity in this regard, but there is evidence that cholesterol is also kept in check by a regular intake of evening primrose oil. The prostaglandins that are formed from the GLA in evening primrose oil also help regulate blood pressure, so some people with high blood pressure may find it begins to drop once they start taking evening primrose oil.

Rheumatoid Arthritis

Recent studies indicate that evening primrose oil can ease the pain and stiffness of rheumatoid arthritis. In this disease the immune system is thought to go awry, and begins to attack itself as it would a foreign invader. Evening primrose oil helps to regulate the immune system so that it can better differentiate between 'friend' and 'foe'. However, whilst evening primrose oil is helpful in rheumatoid arthritis it does seem that even better results are obtained when it is mixed with fish oils.

Mastalgia

A very well respected use of evening primrose oil is in the treatment of benign breast diseases associated with a woman's menstrual cycle. Many doctors now actually recommend or prescribe evening primrose oil for mastalgia. The daily recommended dosage would be around four 500mg capsules but this could be discussed with your doctor.

Hair, Skin and Nails

In a trial that examined the possibility of evening primrose oil as a remedy for dry eyes, it was noted that the condition of skin, hair and nails often improved as well. Many people find evening primrose oil is indeed an internal beauty treatment, making skin softer, nails harder and hair stronger and shinier. In addition the result of the original trial was that evening primrose oil can also help improve dry eyes.

FISH OILS

Mention fish oils and most people think of cod liver oil, which for centuries has been used as a preventative against winter ills.

In 1752, Dr Samuel Kay used cod liver oil at Manchester Infirmary to treat rheumatic pain and bone disorders. Physicians in the Victorian era used cod liver oil to treat gout, consumption, bronchitis, chronic skin diseases and, of course, rickets. While the medics of the time accepted that cod liver oil was effective, no one knew why this was so. Some speculated naïvely that cod liver oil benefited the body by lubricating the joints. It was not until the 'discovery' of vitamins in 1912 that scientists began to understand how and why cod liver oil was of benefit to human health.

It was found to be one of the richest sources of vitamins A and D. By now it had been established that both these vitamins were needed for healthy skin, teeth and gums. It was realized that the reason cod liver oil was so effective against rickets – the debilitating childhood bone disease – was that it provided vitamin D, the lack of which caused the disease. During the Industrial Revolution, rickets was common amongst the children of workers, who spent much of their lives working in appalling conditions.

Because of these discoveries, cod liver oil was regarded as a major player in the growth and development of children. Rickets is normally thought of as a disease of the past, but even today the Department of Health has mounted a campaign to make Asian parents more aware of the risks of rickets and has in fact advocated the use of cod liver oil. In addition to obtaining vitamin D from our diet, we also synthesize it through our skin when exposed to sunlight. Fair-skinned people can just about synthesize this vitamin, but our darker-skinned compatriots find it more difficult to absorb sufficient sunlight to make vitamin D.

Eskimos And Fish Oils
The importance of omega-3 in fish oils was discovered by two Danish scientists, John Dyerberg and Hans Bang, when they accompanied

Dr Hugh Sinclair to Greenland in 1976. Dr Sinclair was the nutritional biochemist who first identified that Eskimos have very low blood cholesterol levels despite a diet which includes the highest animal fat content of any diet in the world.

When Dyerberg and Bang analysed the fats in the Eskimos' blood, they found high levels of the essential fatty acids EPA and DHA. Subsequently there has been consistent interest in the subject, and a number of research papers have been published in medical journals pointing to a connection between omega-3 fatty acids and heart disease. In particular, the EPA content is found to have been most effective in lowering the total blood cholesterol and LDL, and increasing the HDL content.

It was not until the 1970s that scientists realized there was more to fish oils than cod liver oil. Research into the Greenland Eskimos revealed that, despite a diet high in animal fat and protein and low in fibre, the Eskimos had a very low incidence of heart disease and rheumatoid arthritis compared to the rest of the Western world.

At last the magic ingredient behind the generally accepted folklore that fish is good for us, and that it feeds the heart and brain, had been discovered. Its name sounds like something right out of science fiction – omega-3. But omega-3 is far from fiction. It is the name given to a group of essential fatty acids which are derived primarily from oily fish such as mackerel, salmon and herring. They are called 'essential' because the body cannot manufacture them and they must come from the diet. Fish acquire them from algae and phytoplankton.

The omega-3 fatty acids in fish are: eicosapentaenoic (EPA), docosapentaenoic acid (DPA), and docosahexaenoic acid (DHA). The omega-3 fatty acids have been found to have the ability to reduce a group of fats called triglycerides, high levels of which impair the body's ability to break down clots and therefore contribute to the risk of heart attacks (see Chapter 4).

In this context the Eskimo story was particularly interesting for researchers. As a race they rarely suffered heart disease despite a diet of seal and whale blubber, both of which are high in cholesterol. Yet when Eskimos moved to Canada and adopted the same diet as the Canadians, their incidence of heart disease matched that of the native Canadians. It was then found that the influencing factor was the high levels of omega-3s in the Eskimo diet. Since then a number of studies have been carried out which graphically illustrate the effects of fish oils not only on

FISH OILS

Fish oils are rich in polyunsaturated fats,
but of a different family (Omega-3) from those
found in Evening Primrose Oil

The active ingredients are called
EPA and DHA.
(eicosapentaenoic acid)
(docosahexaenoic acid)
EPA is needed for structure of cell wall.
Fish oils also produce beneficial prostaglandins.

Omega-3 family

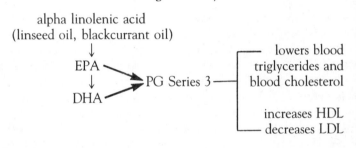

heart health but on arthritis, foetal development, and several skin conditions.

A twenty-year study in Holland (1960–1980), which involved middle-aged men without a history of coronary heart disease, demonstrated that those who consumed at least 1.1 oz. of fish a day had only half the mortality rate from heart attacks as those who ate no fish. A study was set up in Bristol in 1983 to determine whether men who had already suffered a heart attack could reduce the risk of further attacks by a change in their diets. The results demonstrated that men who had increased their consumption of fatty fish had twenty-nine per cent fewer deaths than the group which did not.

Other Conditions That Respond to Fish Oils
The use of fish oil concentrates on sufferers of rheumatoid arthritis has been shown to reduce the symptoms of swollen and tender

joints, morning stiffness and pain. It is believed that the mechanism by which this effect takes place is the suppression of the production of a molecule called leukotriene B4, which has powerful inflammatory properties, as well as the production of interleukin-1, which is involved in the breakdown of cartilage and loss of appetite associated with rheumatoid arthritis.

Another important area of research is the link between essential fatty acids, birthweight and IQ. Babies need both omega-3 and omega-6 (found in vegetable oils) for development. Seventy per cent of human brain cells are made during foetal development, and omega-3 fatty acids are concentrated in the brain. Research has demonstrated that low birthweight babies are deficient in essential fatty acids, and this has been shown to adversely affect the IQ of such children. (See Chapter 3 for further information on foetal development.)

Eczema, acne and psoriasis have also been alleviated by the increase of fish oils in the diet.

Today we eat far less fish, particularly fatty fish like mackerel and herrings – the primary dietary source of omega-3 essential fatty acids. Eskimos consume some 2¹/2 pounds of fatty fish each day (an intake of 6 grams of EPA). Dr Earl Mindell suggests that 'the heart and blood vessels appear to benefit from even minor additions of fish oils to diet; such as three 3 ounce servings of fish (baked, poached or boiled) each week, or 1 gram of fish oil supplement each day.'

Fish Rich in Omega-3 Polyunsaturates

- Mackerel
- Herrings
- Sardines
- Tuna (fresh)
- Lake Trout
- Salmon

Effects of Omega-3 Polyunsaturates

- Reduce the risk of heart disease.
- Reduce the likelihood of blood clot formation.
- Make blood less viscous.
- Improve the immune function and other body systems.

ROYAL JELLY

Cliff Richard, Susan Hampshire and Sebastian Coe all have one thing in common. They all take royal jelly and attest to its very real health-giving properties.

Specifically, these personalities and many other people from different walks of life find that royal jelly gives them the energy they need to fulfil their busy schedules – also that colds and flus are no longer a problem for them (even if everyone else around them is going down with the latest bug), and that generally their health amounts to more than an absence of illness – it is a positive glowing state of health.

Other people, however, have tried royal jelly and found that they can discern no difference whatsoever in their general health, and that the high expense incurred in purchasing the product (it does not come cheap) might as well as have been invested in the Canary Wharf development for all the good it has done.

So what is the truth behind royal jelly? Is it the amazing natural pick-me-up and disease preventer which its marketers claim it to be, or simply a fraud?

Where Does Royal Jelly Come From?

Royal jelly is produced by worker bees for consumption by the queen bee. There are three types of bee in a hive: the queen, the worker and the drone. Worker bees live for about six weeks, cannot reproduce, and perform a variety of tasks in the hive. Drones mate with the queen and live a short life, but the queen bee, who is twice the size of the worker bee, can live for six years and is the reproduction machine for the hive. All three types of bee come from the same type of egg, and for the first three days after laying, the eggs are fed the same type of food. After that the future queen bees are fed on a special diet: the substance which is known as royal jelly.

Not surprisingly, royal jelly seems to be something of a wonder food for bees. The argument rages, however: Is it of any nutritional use to humans?

What Is Royal Jelly?

An analysis of royal jelly shows that it is packed with nutrients. Most of the B vitamins are present (thiamine, riboflavin, nicotinic acid, biotin, inositol, folic acid, pyridoxine, cobalamine, pantothenic acid), together with amino acids (the building blocks of protein), vitamin C, the minerals calcium, potassium, magnesium, phosphorus, sodium, iron, manganese, zinc and cobalt, as well as fatty acids, sugars, hormones and nucleotides. There remains a small percentage of the composition of royal jelly which has still not been identified – and this is considered to be royal jelly's 'magic ingredient' which sets it apart from any other nutritional supplement.

The Health Benefits of Royal Jelly

As stated above, many people find that royal jelly gives them increased stamina and high energy levels. However, royal jelly is reported to have helped in a seemingly endless list of health complaints: from acne, allergies, angina, anorexia, anxiety, and arthritis through to baldness, headaches, herpes, impotence and varicose veins. Generally, if a person does respond to royal jelly, it seems to improve any health complaints they may have.

Fresh or Dried?

Any processing of any nutrient or food will affect its biochemical make-up, and this can be established from its taste. Freeze-dried coffee tastes different from freshly ground and filtered coffee, but still makes a good cup of coffee. Freeze-dried royal jelly is cheaper than fresh royal jelly, but does not seem to produce the same effects as its fresh counterpart.

Does It Work?

Unfortunately to date there have been no clinical trials using royal jelly, and only anecdotal evidence as to its efficacy is available. Still, of the latter there is a copious amount, and it would seem unreasonable to dismiss a supplement simply because no scientific research exists proving its benefit. After all, if Vasco da Gama had taken the same attitude he would have lost even more sailors at sea by refusing to give them limes . . .

At the end of the day, though, as with all supplements, supplementation will only bring benefit if a deficiency of a particular nutrient exists. It would seem reasonable to assume, therefore, that some users of royal jelly have derived no benefit from its alleged powers either because their health is already up to par, or because the causes of their ill-health extend beyond nutritional deficiencies

– namely their whole lifestyle needs to be taken in hand. And if so many people do derive benefit from royal jelly, who would want to take it away from them?

GINSENG

A mysterious and potent herb from the East, ginseng is renowned throughout the world for its alleged aphrodisiac qualities. In the East, however, ginseng has also been used for centuries as a general medicine or, as it is described today, as an 'adaptogen'. Much like royal jelly, ginseng affects different people according to their different ailments, but generally brings the body's functions back into regular working order – like tuning up a car engine. Having said that, there are some definite health benefits derived from taking ginseng: improved stamina and concentration; resistance to stress, disease and fatigue; and protection against radiation.

There are two types of ginseng: panax which is considered to be the genuine article, and eleutheroccus or Siberian ginseng which is botanically different from panax ginseng but which shares the same effects.

Scientific Fact or Anecdotal Evidence?

Unlike royal jelly, there is some documented research on the effects of ginseng. When ginseng was used on members of the US army, it was found to make no difference at all: since army recruits are trained to be at the peak of physical fitness, this merely concurs with the classification of ginseng as an adaptogen. Russian scientists, however, tested ginseng on proofreaders who need good concentration powers with high accuracy and speed. Those using ginseng increased their speed by twelve per cent and decreased mistakes by an amazing fifty-one per cent in comparison with the readers who did not use ginseng. In Sweden, university students undergoing exams were shown to do better when taking ginseng, whilst in this country nurses changing from day to night shifts found that if they took ginseng their problems of moodiness, insomnia and decreased alertness were relieved.

Ginseng appears to stimulate the nervous system, speeding up reflexes and increasing speed and accuracy. Tests have also shown an increase in learning retention. Where ginseng, especially Siberian ginseng, differs from other stimulants such as caffeine is that it does not produce the side effects such as jitteriness; over-stimulation and subsequent exhaustion. Further, ginseng has been shown to reverse and block the effects of alcohol and sedative drugs. Conversely, ginseng also has a calming effect and for this reason is commonly used to alleviate stress. Studies in Korea, Russia, Bulgaria, America and London have all demonstrated the calming effects of ginseng.

However the benefits of ginseng do not end there.

Ginseng: Disease Fighter

A major study involving 60,000 Soviet car workers over several months showed that use of ginseng produced an improvement in general health. Japanese research scientists found that ginseng seems to strengthen the immune system, with all the health benefits which that entails. Hence the benefit of ginseng in recuperation after illness and in the prevention of immune-related diseases, and even in slowing down the ageing process. Ginseng has even been found to help diabetics.

Eat and Drink It?

Ginseng is a root and this is obviously the most potent form in which it can be taken. The traditional method of taking ginseng is to boil the root for between six and ten hours and then drink it as a tea. Alternatively a small piece of the root is chewed until completely soft. Pre-prepared ginseng tea, however, is not medicinally effective. Ginseng root powder tablets or capsules, if a good quality brand, are effective but the best method remains to take it in as raw a form as possible.

In conclusion, ginseng possesses genuinely curative powers which have been substantiated by thousands of years' use and by scientific research. However, it is first and foremost an adaptogen, and benefits will only appear if the body has a need for the special qualities it brings.

SUPEROXIDE DISMUTASE – SOD

As I stated in Chapter 2, free radicals are created when oxygen bonds are broken and cannot stabilize. Whilst free radicals have an important role to play in destroying germs, if they proliferate they have a damaging effect on health. Superoxide dismutase, SOD for short, is an enzyme reputed to rout out free radicals. SOD is produced naturally in the body in the nuclei of cells, but some people do not produce enough SOD. Supplementation with SOD can strengthen the body's immune system and lessen the chances of developing immune-related diseases.

Tests can be undertaken to establish existing levels of SOD, and research is underway to predict how levels will perform. SOD has the ability to reduce lipid peroxides – the heavy-duty free radicals which have a long life and are extremely harmful if present in excess.

SOD is taken either via injections, when it has been shown to be of benefit to sufferers of severe rheumatoid arthritis, Crohn's disease and ulcerative colitis, or via tablets. Unfortunately, whilst tablets are more suitable for general widespread use, when the tablet is swallowed SOD is probably for the most part broken down through the digestive process and therefore rendered inactive. A new process has been developed which is reputed to be active, but in general it would seem that, for the time being, SOD must remain in somewhat restricted use.

LECITHIN

Lecithin is a common ingredient found in many food products, thanks to its ability to combine oil and water-based ingredients. However, lecithin has earned itself a reputation as something of a miracle nutrient, a vital factor in the prevention and treatment of heart disease, and a positive slimming aid.

Lecithin is made by the liver but is also found in egg yolk and was first isolated in 1850. It is also present in soya beans and it is this source which is widely used today. A complex mixture of fats and essential fatty acids, lecithin itself is predominantly fat, combined with phosphorus. The phospholipids in lecithin are linked with choline and inositol, and these are thought to be the active agents in controlling cholesterol and helping the metabolism to burn fat and turn it into energy.

Scientific Studies into Lecithin

Research on laboratory animals has shown that atherosclerosis (hardening of the arteries) can be reversed via the reduction of blood cholesterol and lipids to normal levels. Pure soya bean lecithin, when regularly incorporated into the diet, lowers cholesterol. Lecithin and cholesterol coexist in equilibrium, with lecithin controlling the cholesterol. Being a fat, cholesterol does not mix with water and if left on its own will not pass into the blood but will remain in the arteries, eventually building up deposits there if it is not absorbed. Lecithin, being an emulsifier, can effect absorption of cholesterol into the rest of the body's cells, so avoiding harmful cholesterol deposits.

As an emulsifier, lecithin breaks down fat; large particles of fat act as a landing stage where sticky platelets collect, thereby reducing blood circulation and eventually leading to blood clots. Various studies on sufferers of coronary heart disease have shown low levels of blood lecithin, with a correspondingly increased risk of blood clotting. Further, stickiness of blood platelets is decreased by polyunsaturated fatty acids and linolenic as well as linoleic acid: lecithin is rich in both. This in turn has an effect on the levels of good and bad cholesterol – HDLs and LDLs respectively – by increasing levels of the former and decreasing the latter.

Lecithin as a Slimming Aid

As everyone knows, it is not necessarily how much one eats or what one eats which leads to excess weight. We all know some annoying person who can eat like a horse and stay slender whilst someone else just has to look at a lettuce leaf and put on a stone! The body's metabolism is the reason behind this. Some people have a fast-working metabolism which quickly and efficiently burns energy into fuel, while others have the opposite. Soya lecithin is a phospholipid which emulsifies fat more efficiently and faster than any other nutrient. As an emulsifier, lecithin keeps fat from forming deposits, breaking it up into particles which can be metabolized more easily and thoroughly than large particles; thus lecithin prevents fat build-up.

Finally, lecithin is a natural diuretic so it helps to remove any excess fluid which can contribute to weight gain. Studies have shown that people on a 500-calorie-a-day diet of carbohydrates lost no weight at all, whereas other people on a 1,500-calorie-a-day diet of protein and fat (including lecithin) lost weight. Vegetable oils, incidentally, help the body to build lecithin.

It must be said, however, that calorie restriction is necessary in conjunction with lecithin for weight loss – lecithin won't make you lose weight on a diet of 3,000 calories a day!

GARLIC

The ancient Egyptians would bury their pharaohs with everything deemed necessary to accompany the dead king's spirit into the afterlife. Consequently, gold, servants, and the odd wife or two, were entombed with the pharaoh in his pyramid. As was garlic. (Not garlic itself – that would simply deteriorate – but wood and clay carvings of it.)

Why garlic? you might ask. The ancient Egyptians had discovered the health-giving properties of this special herb and wanted to guarantee the health of the spirit.

An Egyptian papyrus of around 1550 BC includes twenty-two therapeutic recipes using garlic for complaints ranging from bites to heart problems and tumours. And the Egyptians were not alone in their observations of the curative powers of garlic: the Greeks, Romans and Vikings have all left us evidence that garlic was prescribed both as a disease-preventative and as a cure for a variety of illnesses. And Louis Pasteur reported on garlic's anti-bacterial activity in 1858 when he used garlic as an antiseptic. During the two World Wars diluted garlic was used as an antiseptic for wounds and to prevent gangrene.

In this day and age, garlic as a medicinal benefactor has seized the interest of research scientists around the world – so much so that the first World Congress on the Health Significance of Garlic and Garlic Constituents was held in 1990. Amongst the many papers presented at the Congress, one by Dr Robert Lin suggested that a daily dose of garlic and garlic extract can substantially reduce the risk of cancer and cardiovascular disease.

Nutrition Research (1987) published the results of a study into the effect of garlic on cholesterol levels. Thirty-two subjects with high levels of cholesterol were split into two groups: one group was given four capsules of liquid garlic extract daily, the other a placebo. Blood levels were measured each month. At first cholesterol levels rose in the garlic takers – probably because garlic shifts lipids (fats) from the tissues, where it has been stored, into the blood where it can be dealt with. After three months of the trial, levels of fatty deposits (lipids) began to fall, reaching normal levels after six months. In 1990 the German Association of General Practitioners from thirty different centres and involving 261 patients conducted a four-month study into the effect of concentrated garlic powder capsules on both cholesterol and triglyceride levels. Results showed a reduction of triglyceride levels by seventeen per cent and of cholesterol levels by twelve per cent. Ten other clinical trials showed that concentrated garlic powder tablets can reduce cholesterol levels by eleven per cent and triglycerides by thirteen per cent.

Garlic: Liquid, Powdered or Aged?

The garlic used in clinical trials is obviously different from the garlic bulbs which we buy for cooking use, although their essence is the same. When you buy garlic it is odourless, and its pungent smell is only released when it is crushed or cut. Each of garlic's cells contains, among other elements, an amino acid, alliin, and an enzyme, allinase. When a clove is cut the amino acid and the enzyme fuse to produce a new substance, allicin, which has a pungent odour. Allicin is very unstable and oxidizes at temperatures above 4°C into many sulphur-based compounds. It is this unique spectrum of sulphur-containing nutrients that give garlic its health-giving properties.

Traditional Chinese herbalists used garlic cloves which had been aged for two to three years in vinegar for numerous health complaints. Today, garlic is aged by slicing it (without using heat) and leaving it in stainless steel tanks for approximately twenty months. During this 'cold-ageing' time, as it is known, the alliin is converted via allicin to a whole host of new beneficial garlic compounds, so that cold-aged garlic is reputed to have more health benefits than ordinary garlic preparations. The end product of the cold-ageing process is completely odourless – a definite plus point for anyone who isn't a hermit! Cold-aged garlic is available in liquid form and dried tablet form.

How Does Garlic Improve Cardiovascular Health?

Cardiovascular health is at risk if high blood pressure, high cholesterol levels and high platelet stickiness exist. Garlic affects all three of these factors beneficially and consequently lessens the risk of heart disease, providing of course that a reasonably healthy lifestyle is maintained.

A heart attack occurs when a blood clot forms in one of the arteries leading to the heart. Blood clots are formed when platelets build up and become trapped with red blood cells in fibrin, which is a mesh-like substance. Platelets are tiny blood cells which control the rate at which blood clots. High cholesterol levels, smoking, stress and numerous other factors make the platelets stickier, and consequently slow down blood flow. Garlic extract reduces platelet stickiness thanks to its ajoene, an anticlotting factor.

Garlic also appears to lower high blood pressure, perhaps by having a dilatory effect on the blood vessels, so reducing pressure. Whatever the (as yet unascertained) reason, trials on 100 patients with abnormally high blood pressure showed a significant reduction in the blood pressure of forty people, after just one week's dosage of garlic. Chinese herbalists have used garlic to relieve high blood pressure for many years and it is a part of their standard practice.

Garlic reduces cholesterol levels, and also levels of triglycerides. As explained in Chapter 4, not all fats are harmful, and some are necessary for human health. Low density lipoproteins (LDLs) are considered to be injurious to health, whilst high density lipoproteins (HDLs) protect against heart attacks and strokes. Numerous tests have shown that garlic increases levels of HDLs and lowers those of LDLs.

The Anti-Infection Effects of Garlic

Garlic's sulphur compounds are antifungal and antibacterial, which makes it effective in numerous health problems. Garlic helps fight against colds and flu since it is an antioxidant and strengthens the immune system; and it also makes short shrift of diarrhoea, tummy upsets, and the yeast syndrome.

Garlic as a Preventative Medicine

People who take garlic capsules from September to March often find that they escape the winter round of colds and flu, or that colds are shorter and less severe. At the same time, of course, cardiovascular health is maintained.

Garlic boosts the immune system seemingly by increasing the number of white blood cells – the body's defence army. Also, the sulphur compounds in garlic protect against free radicals which if left unchecked are hazardous to health (more about this in Chapter 2).

In summary, garlic is no mythical cure best left to ward off vampires. Its medicinal properties have been recognized since ancient times by many different civilizations. Only from the mid-nineteenth century did we begin to discover how garlic achieves what it does, and only in this century have the links between garlic and heart health and the immune system become clearer. Who knows what other health benefits of this remarkable herb will come to light over the next decade?

Conclusion

The 'wonder nutrients' are not magic pills and potions which by themselves can ensure our good health no matter what harmful substances we present to our bodies. Further, if the body already has an adequate supply of a nutrient, it will do no good to supplement with that nutrient as the body will either pass the surplus out of its system or store it for later use (with possible toxic consequences).

Garlic, evening primrose oil, royal jelly, ginseng and lecithin all have definite nutrients present in their make-up which account for their efficacy – these are not quack medicines. In fact, the ancient lore of garlic for colds, ginseng for relaxation, and so on, is now being substantiated by scientific studies and is being recognized as far more than superstition and mumbo jumbo.

What is more, unlike chemical drugs which have unpleasant side effects, these 'wonder nutrients' are safe and a good deal more natural (however much they may have been processed from their original herbs and roots) than their drug counterparts, and their use over the centuries has long demonstrated their efficacy.

7

Choosing a Supplement

Ignorance solves no problems
Disraeli (1804–1881)

IN AN IDEAL world supplementation would be unneccessary, but while we should strive for the ideal, we also need to be realistic. The overwhelming message from experts is that food alone is not enough.

It is not enough because the nutritional quality of our food can only be as good as the quality of the soil in which it is grown, or the grasses upon which the animals graze. It is not enough because, however nutrient-packed the original product, refining, storing, processing, freezing, and even air, all play their part in depleting essential nutrients. It is not enough because each individual has his or her own nutritional requirements, some of which may exceed the amount that could possibly be ingested from even the healthiest of diets.

In addition, as we have seen, there are the ravages of stress, illness, pollution and the extra demands of young children, and pregnant or breastfeeding mothers.

Supplementation offers us a realistic approach which can help guarantee optimal nutrient intake which food alone cannot. A wholesome diet plus supplements is a realistic approach to optimum health.

This interest in nutrition and diet has also created increasing confusion on the subject of the type and quantity of supplements. It has given rise to a plethora of pills, potions and powders all with health-giving properties. Enter a health food store, pharmacy, or even the supermarket, and you will be confronted by hundreds of bottles filled with tablets, capsules and powders. So which one best meets your needs? To confound you even further, the labels do not simply give the nutrient name, such as vitamin C or iron, but also such terms as 'chelated', 'timed-release', 'divided dose' and 'high potency'. What does it all mean?

WHICH SUPPLEMENT?

A *Multivitamin and Mineral Supplement*
A well-balanced multivitamin and mineral preparation may be all that a person needs. Alternatively it can form the basis of a regime in which extra single nutrients are added for those with specific needs. Chosen wisely, it can provide a proper balance of nutrients, and is the ideal choice unless individual nutrients have been prescribed by a nutritionist or a doctor.

A basic multivitamin and mineral preparation should contain at least the following nutrients: Vitamin A, beta carotene, B complex, vitamin C, vitamin D, vitamin E, phosphorus, calcium, magnesium, potassium, iron, zinc, manganese, copper, iodine, molybdenum, chromium, selenium, and vanadium.

A superior multivitamin and mineral preparation would also contain additional nutrients such as: choline, inositol, methionine, PABA, bioflavonoids, lysine, lecithin, rutin, betaine, hesperdine and cysteine.

High Potency Vitamins
More is not necessarily better. Most vitamins and minerals work in the body in conjunction with enzymes. The body has a maximum capacity for production of each enzyme – so only a certain amount of a vitamin or mineral can be used in accordance with the availability of that enzyme. In most cases consuming more than the required amount will not increase the metabolic activity. Instead the body will either store the excess nutrient if it is fat soluble (for example, vitamins A and D) or will flush it out if it is water soluble (for example, vitamin C).

Megadoses of the fat soluble vitamins A and D over long periods of time can produce toxic effects and can also interfere with the absorption and use of other nutrients.

Timed-Release Supplements
'Timed-release', 'continuous action', and 'sustained release' are synonymous terms denoting a process whereby the ingredients of

a tablet are trickled out of a binding matrix. In contrast to a conventional tablet, which releases all of the ingredients within a short period of time, timed-release tablets release small quantities over a prolonged period, a process particularly useful in the case of water-soluble vitamins.

Chelated Minerals
A chelated mineral is one that is chemically bound to another substance; in nature this is usually a protein or group of amino acids. Although research is as yet inconclusive, it is generally accepted that amino acid chelates are absorbed in far greater amounts than any other mineral form. Their absorption is at least three times and, in some cases up to ten times, the amount of non-chelated forms.

'Natural' and 'Organic'
The words 'natural' and 'organic' have little to offer in the case of supplements except to increase the cost. The process of extracting nutrients from foods can hardly be termed 'natural', and in many cases chemical solvents are used to extract the nutrients.

DOSAGES

Bioavailability

This term refers to the amount of an ingested nutrient that is absorbed and utilized by the body. Just swallowing a multivitamin supplement does not mean that a person will benefit from the full quantity of the nutrients in the pill. Unless the nutrients are consumed in optimal ratios to other nutrients there will not be the maximum absorption from the digestive tract into the bloodstream. Additionally, the nutrient must be ingested in a form that the body can convert for use in the metabolic process. Poorly made supplements may even pass through the body without even dissolving.

The bioavailability of a supplement is affected by other dietary components. For example, a high intake of fibre will inhibit calcium absorption, while supplementing the diet with large amounts of iron or zinc may inhibit the absorption of some trace minerals. This is because the minerals compete with each other for absorption – when one is provided in abundance, a secondary deficiency of another mineral may result.

Overdosing and Toxicity

Too much of anything can be harmful. Even water can kill if taken in excess. Vitamins and minerals are amongst the safest substances that one can take, and in order for them to be toxic one would have to take enormous quantities.

A compound is said to be toxic when it destroys chemical reactions in the body which then result in new symptoms and signs; these are sometimes termed as 'side effects.' The degree of toxicity of any compound is determined by its molecules. A vast majority of modern drugs are made up of xenobiotic molecules, which are not normally found in the body. In contrast, nutrients such as vitamins are orthomolecules and have been present in the body since life began. The body is therefore familiar with orthomolecules and has developed ways of disposing of them when they are present in excess. As for the xenobiotics, the body has to use enzymes to detoxify itself of them and this results in interference with enzyme reactions. Therefore, the danger of side effects from vitamins and other nutrients is far smaller than with most modern drugs.

In ideal circumstances, a perfect therapeutic molecule should cure without side effects. As the perfect molecule does not exist, however, one has to look for the least imperfect molecule. Orthomolecules are less imperfect than xenobiotics. However, as vitamin therapies have gained in popularity, the reservations expressed by xenobiotics practitioners have been reflected by the popular media. It has been claimed that vitamin deficiency is not all that common in this country and that supplementation is therefore a waste. What is more significant is the claim that concentrated doses of vitamins can be dangerous and even lethal. Primarily the danger is seen in the use of megavitamin therapy, that is, the use of massive doses of some forms of vitamins, such as B3.

The general definition of a megadose is a dose of the nutrient at least ten times the average Recommended Daily Allowance (RDA). Megavitamins have been found necessary when the body is unable to absorb adequate quantities of vitamins in the stomach, or in certain cases where vitamins do not function properly in the body. As any substance can be harmful in excess, every consumer should consider the safety of using vitamins as drugs.

It seems ironic that while modern medicine finds justification for the use of highly toxic radiation and chemotherapy for cancer treatment, it raises such a hue and cry about the toxicity of vitamins and other nutrients. Obviously something else is bothering the opponents of orthomolecular medicine . . .

Disgruntled with the National Health Service, more and more people in Britain are turning to alternative therapies despite the fact that they have to pay for the privilege. Recent drug scandals, like those concerning Opren and even aspirin, have made the public much more conscious of the dangers of xenobiotics. In America too, while professional health care (perhaps more appropriately termed professional disease care) is widely available, because of the increasing cost of such modern medical care more and more Americans are turning to self-help remedies. It is not surprising therefore, to meet with an adverse reaction from the practitioners whose very livelihood has been threatened as these self-help remedies continue to make the public less reliant on the medical profession, not to mention the pharmaceutical barons.

Whatever the case, in order to form an independent opinion on the therapeutic value of any substance, the possibility of adverse effects and toxicity must be considered. So, as the consumer is faced with a wide choice of vitamin and mineral products, who does he turn to? Naturally, the first recourse is the GP, but most physicians have had little or no training in nutrition sciences. The next traditional source is the pharmacist, but once again, his exposure to information on nutrition has been minimal during his formal training.

Nutritionists, dietitians and health counsellors may be alternative sources of information and therapy. There are thousands of health food shop staff who may, in varying degrees, be able to assist, and who, in contrast to the 'disease professionals', are able to provide advice on balanced diets, proper nutrition and supplementation. There has so far been little recognition either by the medical profession or the government, of the valuable contribution these 'real health professionals' make to the health of the nation, so it is encouraging to note that the public, at least, has recognized their worth.

VITAMINS: HOW SAFE?

- **Vitamin B1 – Thiamin**
  There are very few reports of adverse reactions to thiamin in medical literature. Thiamin is generally considered to be safe and non-toxic when taken by mouth; injections have resulted in a few allergic reactions, but life-threatening situations are rarely encountered.
- **Vitamin B2 – Riboflavin**
  Riboflavin is not considered to be toxic, and excess riboflavin is rapidly passed out of the body via the urine.
- **Vitamin B3 – Niacin**
  No real toxic effects of niacin are known. However, large doses (over 500mg per day) can cause side effects such as a tingling sensation, flushing of the skin, gastro-intestinal distress, and glucose intolerance.
- **Vitamin B5 – Pantothenic Acid**
  Pantothenic acid is thought to be non-toxic. Excessive doses as large as 10,000mg per day have produced no known adverse effects.
- **Vitamin B6 – Pyridoxine**
  The toxicity of B6 is extremely low and is non-toxic up to 100mg per day. However people taking 200mg or more per day for long periods may become dependent on the vitamin.
- **Vitamin B12 – Cyanocobolamine**
  Vitamin B12 is considered non-toxic.
- **Vitamin H – Biotin**
  Biotin is generally non-toxic in humans.
- **Folic Acid**
  Folic acid is considered to be non-toxic to man.
- **Vitamin C – Ascorbic Acid**
  Clinical trials, using over seven thousand volunteers who received up to 30g of vitamin C a day, revealed vey few problems.
- **Vitamin A**
  Symptoms of vitamin A toxicity have been observed in adults ingesting in excess of 50,000i.u. a day for several years.
- **Vitamin D**
  Popularly called the 'sun' vitamin. The maximum dietary intake of vitamin D usually accepted as sensible is 1000i.u.
- **Vitamin E – Tocopherol**
  This is the least toxic of the fat-soluble vitamins. A high intake of vitamin E may increase the need for other fat-soluble vitamins.

PART TWO
THE HEALTH ESSENTIALS
NUTRIENT GUIDE

8

Recommended Nutrient Intakes

STANDARDS IN THE FORM of Recommended Intakes for Nutrients and Recommended Daily Amounts (RDA) of food energy and nutrients have existed in the UK for over thirty years.

In order to update them in the light of more recent information, the Department of Health's Chief Medical Officer asked the Committee on Medical Aspects of Food Policy (COMA) to set up a panel of experts to consider the matter. The panel revised the standards and came up with the following new standards.

Estimated Average Requirement (EAR)   The panel's estimate of the average requirement or need for food energy or a nutrient. Clearly, many people will need more than the average, and many people will need less.

Reference Nutrient Intake (RNI)   An amount of a nutrient that is enough for almost every individual, even someone who has high needs for the nutrient. This level of intake is, therefore, considerably higher than most people need. If individuals are consuming the RNI of a nutrient they are most unlikely to be deficient in that nutrient. RNIs are equivalent in definition to the old RDAs.

Lower Reference Nutrient Intake (LRNI)   The amount of a nutrient that is enough for only the small number of people with low needs. Most people will need more than the LRNI if they are to eat enough. If individuals are habitually eating less than the LRNI they will almost certainly be deficient.

Safe Intake   A term normally used to indicate the intake of a nutrient for which there is not enough information to estimate requirements. A safe intake is one which is judged to be adequate for almost everyone's needs but not so large as to cause undesirable effects.

MAJOR RECOMMENDATIONS ON DIET

Energy

The energy needs of British people as estimated by the COMA panel are shown in the box below.

The figures for energy were based on present low activity levels. There was broad agreement that an increase in energy expenditure was necessary for the population as a whole, which if achieved would mean an increase in the figures.

Estimated Average Requirements for Energy (kcal/day)

Age	Males	Females
0–3 months	545	515
4–6 months	690	645
7–9 months	825	765
10–12 months	920	865
1–3 years	1,230	1,165
4–6 years	1,715	1,545
7–10 years	1,970	1,740
11–14 years	2,220	1,845
15–18 years	2,755	2,110
19–50 years	2,550	1,940
51–59 years	2,500	1,900
60–64 years	2,380	1,900
65–74 years	2,330	1,900
75+ years	2,110	1,810

Carbohydrates

The recommendations of the committee were that about 37% of the energy content of the diet should come from starches, intrinsic sugars (sugars in fruits) and lactose (milk sugar). Anybody obtaining less than around 37% of their energy from these carbohydrate sources was probably relying too heavily on fat and protein as an energy source.

It was felt by the panel that no more than 10% of the energy content of the diet should be derived from extrinsic sugars (for instance, sweets and confectionery), as above that level there were attendant risks of dental caries and so on.

Fibre

The panel proposed that the average intake of fibre should be 18 g/day in adults, with an expected range of individual intakes from 12–24g depending on body size.

Protein

The 1991 COMA figures for protein are quite a bit lower than previous recommendations. This is because figures have previously been based on average protein intakes rather than on how much the body actually needs.

It was felt that the maximum protein intake for a normal person should not exceed twice the RNI. The exception may be very active people or those engaged in strength sports.

Fat

The panel decided that the specific types of fat eaten were more important than the total fat consumed. Hence it is conceivable that someone with a higher total fat intake could be at less health risk than someone with a lower total fat intake – purely because of a difference in the types of fat eaten.

- The total fat content of the diet should on average provide 33% of the total energy intake.
- No more than 10% of the total energy intake should come from saturated fatty acids.
- Approximately 6% of the total energy intake should come from polyunsaturated fatty acids.
- Approximately 12% of the total energy intake should come from monounsaturated fatty acids.

- Trans-fatty acids (found in heat processed oils) should provide no more than 2% of the total energy intake.

The COMA Recommendations on Fat

Age	(g/day)	Age	(g/day)
0–3 months	12.5	15–18 years (males)	55.2
4–6 months	12.7	15–18 years (females)	45.4
7–9 months	13.7	19–49 years (males)	55.5
10–12 months	14.9	19–49 years (females)	45.0
1–3 years	14.5	50+ years (males)	53.3
4–6 years	19.7	50+ years (females)	46.5
7–10 years	28.3	Pregnancy	51.0
11–14 years (males)	42.1	Lactation (0–6 months)	56.0
11–14 years (females)	41.2	(6+ months)	53.0

Vitamins and Minerals

The 1991 COMA report also details recommendations for daily intakes of many vitamins and minerals. These are dealt with separately in the following chapter.

9

A Directory of Vitamins and Minerals

VITAMIN A

K NOWN AS THE vision vitamin, for its role in eyesight, this was the first vitamin to be discovered. Vitamin A is one of the fat-soluble vitamins and as such can be stored in the liver. In ancient Egypt, the cure for poor eyesight was to eat raw liver. Low levels of this nutrient can cause night blindness, and it is essential for vision in dim light. In the developing world where vitamin A deficiency is very severe, mega dosages of around 300,000i.u. are given to children on a yearly or six-monthly basis. Sadly, despite this, around a quarter of a million children in the world still become blind through vitamin A deficiency each year.

What Does It Do?

- Maintains healthy skin and mucous membranes – helping to protect against infection of the nose, throat, lungs, urinary tract etc.
- Necessary in the formation of visual purple, an eye pigment involved in night vision.
- Needed for proper development of the foetus in the womb.
- Influences proper bone development.

Signs of Deficiency

Severe vitamin A deficiency leads to various physical changes in the eye and eventually leads to blindness. A marginal vitamin A deficiency will lead to increased susceptibility to respiratory tract infections and skin problems.

How Much?

The RNI Values (COMA 1991) for Vitamin A

Age	(mcg/day)	(i.u./day)	Age	(mcg/day)	(i.u./day)
0–12 months	350	1,167	11–14 years (male)	600	2,000
1–6 years	400	1,333	15+ years (male)	700	2,333
7–10 years	500	1,667	Pregnancy	700	2,333
11+ years (female)	600	2,000	Lactation	950	3,167

Food Sources

The main food sources of vitamin A in the diet are liver, carrots, milk, margarine and butter.

Food	Retinol (mcg/100g)	(i.u./100g)	Food	Retinol (mcg/100g)	(i.u./100g)
Halibut liver oil	900,000	3,000,000	Eggs	190	633
Lamb's liver	19,900	66,333	Pig's kidney	160	533
Cod liver oil	18,000	60,000	Milk	56	187
Butter	985	3,283	Mackerel	45	150
Margarine	800	2,667	Beef	10	33
Cheese, cheddar	363	1,210	Sardines, canned	7	23

Reasons To Supplement

Vitamin A can be taken by anyone who is worried that they may be at risk of marginal vitamin A deficiency. This could include:

- Vegetarians.
- Diabetics (who cannot efficiently convert beta carotene into vitamin A).

- Those with fat malabsorption syndrome.
- Those with other impaired absorption conditions (for instance, coeliacs or gastrectomy patients).
- Those with feverish states or kidney conditions which may cause excessive amounts of vitamin A to be lost from the body.

Vitamin A has also been used successfully in the treatment of certain skin conditions, for example, acne and psoriasis.

How Safe?

Vitamin A is one of the vitamins that if taken in excess can lead to toxicity because it is stored in the liver. However, it still has a high safety margin in that regular daily intakes generally have to exceed 7,500mcg (25,000i.u.) in women, and 9,000mcg (30,000i.u.) in men, before toxic side effects are experienced.

The vitamin A intake of pregnant women, or women likely to become pregnant should not exceed 3,300mcg (11,000i.u.) per day (combined from food and supplements) unless directed.

The effects of vitamin A excess would take the form of skin scaling, joint pains, liver enlargement and nausea. Vitamin A toxicity is usually fully reversible.

Interactions With Other Substances

Vitamin A and vitamin D are found together in many food sources, although they are not actually dependent upon one another for their absorption or utilization.

A deficiency of the mineral zinc can affect the function of vitamin A and vice versa. Vitamin A should not be taken with vitamin A derivative acne drugs.

BETA CAROTENE

Beta carotene, derived from vegetable sources is sometimes referred to as provitamin A. It is found in plant foods and basically consists of two vitamin A molecules joined end to end. This nutrient is found in the yellow or orange pigment present in many fruits and vegetables. The human body can readily convert beta carotene into vitamin A.

It was as early as 1830 that the yellow pigment in carrots was isolated and named 'carotene'. However, until 1919 the connection between carotene and vitamin A was not known and it took a further thirty-two years to establish the differences in the structure of the two nutrients.

It is now known that people with high levels of beta carotene in their diets have less chance of developing certain types of cancers than those with a lower intake of the nutrient.

International Units (i.u.s) of beta carotene should not be confused with i.u.s of vitamin A activity. (Only i.u.s of vitamin A, have scientific meaning.) I.u.s of beta carotene divided by three gives i.u.s of vitamin A activity, so a traditionally labelled 25,000i.u. (15mg) beta carotene supplement will provide the body with 8,333i.u. of vitamin A.

What Does It Do?

In addition to all the functions of vitamin A, beta carotene is thought to be a free radical quencher. This means it has the capacity to protect delicate cell contents from damage and possibly inactivates mutagens and carcinogens.

Signs of Deficiency

Deficiency symptoms of beta carotene are the same as those for vitamin A.

How Much?

Dietary beta carotene contributes towards total vitamin A intake. There is deemed to be no separate requirement for beta carotene.

Reasons To Supplement

Beta carotene may be taken purely for its vitamin A activity, but the nutrient's free radical quenching capacity also makes it a useful supplement in other respects.

Many studies now show that low intakes of beta carotene are

associated with the development of cancer and heart disease. With this in mind, nutrition experts underline the importance of taking two to three good portions of fruit and vegetables daily. If this sort of dietary level is not being achieved, a supplement of beta carotene may be advisable.

Beta carotene supplementation is also recommended before prolonged exposure to hot sun. It can help to protect the skin from u.v. induced damage and may even protect against skin cancer in the long term.

Another possible use for beta carotene is to help lessen any side effects experienced during radiation therapy.

NB: The Medicines Act 1968 strictly prohibits any product being recommended for cancer treatment.

Food Sources

Beta carotene providing Vitamin A			Beta carotene providing Vitamin A		
Food	(mcg/100g)	(i.u./100g)	Food	(mcg/100g)	(i.u./100g)
Carrots (old)	12,000	6,667	Mango	1,200	667
Spinach	6,000	3,333	Tomatoes	600	333
Sweet potato	4,000	2,233	Cabbage	300	167
Apricots, dried	3,600	2,000	Peas, frozen	300	167
Watercress	3,000	1,667	Potatoes	0	0

How Safe?

Beta carotene is an extremely safe form of taking vitamin A, because at very high levels of beta carotene intake, the body's beta-carotene-to-vitamin-A conversion process slows down dramatically.

The only known side effect occurring with high levels of beta carotene is 'carotenaemia' which is a harmless condition in which the skin turns a slightly orange colour. This is reversible upon stopping beta carotene supplementation. Carotenaemia may occur at dosages of approximately 30mg daily and above.

Interactions With Other Substances

Beta carotene cannot be properly converted into vitamin A by diabetics or those with hypothyroidism or severe liver malfunctioning.

These people should therefore not rely on beta carotene as a source of vitamin A activity.

THE B VITAMINS

The B vitamins are an interrelated group of water-soluble nutrients. Also called B-complex, they occur together in foods. They are B1 thiamin, B2 riboflavin, B3 niacin, B5 pantothenic acid, B6 pyridoxine, biotin, folic acid, and B12 cyanocobalamin. These are true vitamins. For a substance to qualify as a true vitamin it must satisfy three conditions.

- It cannot be made by the body and must come from food.
- Deficiency of the substance produces clinical symptoms.
- By administering the substance, symptoms and signs of deficiency can be reversed.

The other members of the B family are choline, inositol and para-aminobenzoic acid.

Jointly they are responsible for the maintenance of the nervous system, good mental health, and efficient digestion.

- Stress increases the body's requirement for the B vitamins.
- The milling process of white flour removes five of the B vitamins.
- Thiamin (B1), riboflavin (B2) and niacin are collectively referred to as 'energy vitamins'.
- Biotin and pantothenic acid (B5) are known as the 'anti-stress vitamins'.
- Pyridoxine (B6) is often called the 'anti-depression vitamin'.

THIAMIN

Thiamin is also known as vitamin B1 and was first isolated from rice polishings in 1926 as the factor that prevented beri-beri. It was the first B vitamin to be named and numbered. The main cause of thiamin deficiency is alcoholism. Thiamin is one of the vitamins most easily attacked by environmental conditions. It is water soluble and is lost by leaching into cooking water or dripping from thawed frozen foods. It is also destroyed rapidly by alkalis (for example, bicarbonate of soda), and ultra-violet light. The preservative sulphur dioxide also destroys thiamin.

What Does It Do?

Thiamin functions in the body as part of the coenzyme thiamin pyrophosphate. This coenzyme is vital for the release of energy from carbohydrates, fats and alcohol.

Signs of Deficiency

A severe deficiency of thiamin is now rarely seen in the West, but extremely low intakes lead to a condition known as beri-beri, which is fatal if not quickly treated with thiamin. Symptoms of beri-beri are muscle weakness, nausea, a loss of appetite, and water retention leading to heart and lung damage.

Minor thiamin deficiencies are known to cause mental conditions such as depression, irritability, lack of concentration and memory loss. Loss of weight and gastro-intestinal upsets are also noted.

How Much?

The RNI Values (COMA 1991) for Thiamin

Age	(mg/day)	Age	(mg/day)
0–9 months	0.2	15–18 years (males)	1.1
10–12 months	0.3	15+ years (females)	0.8
1–3 years	0.5	19–50 years (males)	1.0
4–10 years	0.7	50+ years (males)	0.9
11–14 years (females)	0.7	Pregnancy (last trimester)	0.9
11–14 years (males)	0.9	Lactation	1.0

It must be noted that these figures are for people with very low levels of physical activity both at work and at leisure. More active people would need correspondingly more thiamin.

Food Sources

Food	Thiamin (mg/100g)	Food	Thiamin (mg/100g)
Yeast extract	3.1	Peanuts, roasted	0.23
Fortified breakfast cereal	1.8	Bread, white	0.21
Soya beans, dry	1.10	Potatoes	0.2
Pork chop	0.57	Chicken	0.11
Rice	0.41	Beef, stewing steak	0.06
Bread, wholemeal	0.34	Milk	0.05
Peas, frozen	0.32		

The main sources of thiamin in the diet are bread and cereal products, potatoes, milk and meat.

Reasons To Supplement

Thiamin may be taken in supplement form to guard against any possibility of a deficiency.

Factors that increase the need for thiamin are:
- High carbohydrate intake.
- High alcohol intake.
- Habitual antacid or barbiturate use.
- Physical or mental stress.

A blood test is capable of revealing a state of thiamin deficiency with precision, and clinical experience has found that positive tests are particularly common in emotionally unstable individuals who have sometimes received psychotherapy for years without benefit.

It is also well known that alcoholics frequently become thiamin deficient, and large doses of the vitamin can be very beneficial to such individuals.

All in all, thiamin has been recorded as being effective in more than 230 diseases. However, this has given rise to scepticism on the basis that such a 'cure-all' could not exist. Nevertheless, some of the conditions that have been successfully treated with thiamin are lumbago, sciatica, trigeminal neuralgia, facial paralysis and optic neuritis.

Taken as a supplement, thiamin is also reported to deter insect bites.

How Safe?

Long-term intakes of up to 3,000mg/day have not caused undesirable side effects in adults.

Interactions With Other Substances

It is usually recognized that B vitamins are best taken together for most general purposes. However there is no detriment in taking thiamin singly for a specific reason.

RIBOFLAVIN

Riboflavin (vitamin B2) is a member of the B-complex which is naturally a bright yellow colour. It was isolated from whey by Dr Khun in 1933. Riboflavin is a yellow-green compound that is soluble in water but not in fats. Meat and milk are the main sources of riboflavin, and therefore vegans are at the greatest risk of deficiency.

Riboflavin is relatively unaffected by cooking processes, but is destroyed by alkalis (for instance, bicarbonate of soda), and exposure to light – thus milk left on the doorstep will lose all its B2 content.

What Does It Do?

Riboflavin forms the essential coenzymes FAD (flavin dinucleotide) and FMN (flavin mononucleotide). These two are essential for converting proteins, fats and carbohydrates into energy in the presence of oxygen.

Signs of Deficiency

Typically, deficiency symptoms take the form of oral complaints such as sore burning lips and tongue ailments. An oily-type dermatitis is also often present down either side of the nose. Eyes can also be affected, with burning, itchiness and visual fatigue present.

How Much?

The RNI Values (COMA 1991) for Riboflavin

Age	(mg/day)	Age	(mg/day)
0–12 months	0.4	11+ years (females)	1.1
1–3 years	0.6	15+ years (males)	1.3
4–6 years	0.8	Pregnancy	1.4
7–10 years	1.0	Lactation	1.6
11–14 years (males)	1.2		

Food Sources

Food	Riboflavin (mg/100g)	Food	Riboflavin (mg/100g)
Yeast extract	11.0	Cheese, cheddar	0.5
Lamb's liver	4.64	Eggs	0.47
Pig's kidney	2.58	Beef, stewing steak	0.23
Fortified breakfast cereal	1.6	Milk	0.17
Wheatgerm	0.61	Chicken	0.13

The main sources of riboflavin in the diet are milk, meat, fortified cereal products and eggs.

Reasons To Supplement

Riboflavin supplementation is necessary in those with a deficiency of this nutrient. Such a deficiency is not uncommon in people who have undergone total or partial gastrectomy, and in those being treated with chloramphenicol or other antibiotics.

In high amounts, riboflavin has been reported to be of use in eye conditions such as blepharitis (sore itchy eyelids) and keratitis (inflammation of the cornea). Riboflavin is also occasionally effective in the treatment of migraines and muscle cramps, but there is no known rationale for this.

How Safe?

Intakes of more than 120 mg/day for ten months have not been associated with any adverse side effects. Absorption of riboflavin from the intestine is limited by poor solubility and so it is unlikely that enough could be absorbed to be harmful.

Interactions With Other Substances

It is usually recognized that B vitamins are best taken together for most general purposes. However there is no detriment in taking riboflavin singly for a specific reason.

Thiazide diuretics can increase the excretion of riboflavin.

Riboflavin is unstable in the presence of the antibiotics erythromycin and tetracycline. The vitamin should be taken apart from these drugs.

Riboflavin may affect the way cancer cells respond to the anticancer drug methotrexate.

NB: Riboflavin supplements may cause a harmless yellow coloration of the urine.

NIACIN

Two related compounds – nicotinic acid and niacinamide (nicotinamide) – are both called niacin. Niacin is also commonly known as vitamin B3, the vitamin that prevents the deficiency disease pellagra. A first cure for pellagra was a diet of yeast, meat and milk, yet it was not known until much later that this was because of a high level of nicotinic acid. Niacin, like all the other B vitamins, is water soluble.

In addition to pre-formed niacin occurring in foods, niacin may also be made in the body from the essential amino acid tryptophan. However this conversion is very inefficient, with sixty molecules of tryptophan needed to make one molecule of niacin. (The exception is pregnant women, where the conversion is twice as efficient.)

The conversion of tryptophan to niacin also requires the presence of other nutrients such as thiamin, pyridoxine (vitamin B6), and biotin.

Niacin is one of the most stable of the B vitamins, being unaffected by light, air or alkalis. The only appreciable loss of niacin occurs when it leaches into cooking water.

What Does It Do?

The two forms of niacin – nicotinic acid and nicotinamide – have different functions. The acid form is concerned with the blood circulation, maintenance of the nervous system, and the reduction of cholesterol and fats. The amide form, nicotinamide, assists in the breakdown of carbohydrates, fats and protein, and energy production.

Niacin forms two coenzymes in the body, namely nicotinamide adenine dinucleotide (NAD) and nicotinamide adenine dinucleotide phosphate (NADP). These coenzymes, like the ones formed by thiamin and riboflavin, are involved in the release of energy from food.

How Much?

*The RNI Values (COMA 1991) for Niacin Equivalent**

Age	(mg/day)	Age	(mg/day)
0–6 months	3	15–18 years (females)	14
7–9 months	4	15–18 years (male)	18
10–12 months	5	19–50 years (female)	13
1–3 years	8	19–50 years (male)	17
4–6 years	11	50+ years (female)	12
7–10 years	12	50+ years (male)	16
11–14 years (females)	12	Lactation	15
11–14 years (males)	15		

* Niacin equivalent≈ available niacin + (tryptophan : 60)

Signs of Deficiency

The disease pellagra results from a deficiency of niacin, and is characterized by the three D's – diarrhoea, dermatitis and dementia. Pellagra will eventually lead to death if not treated with niacin. Symptoms of a more minor niacin deficiency are tiredness, depression and loss of memory.

Food Sources

The main sources of niacin in the diet are meat and meat products, potatoes, bread and fortified breakfast cereals.

Food	Niacin	Tryptophan	Niacin equiv.		Niacin	Tryptophan	Niacin equiv.
Coffee,				Fish, white	2.9	189	6.0
instant	24.8	186	27.9	Mung beans,			
Chicken	5.9	221	9.6	dry	2.0	210	5.5
Beef,				Eggs	0.1	217	3.7
Stewing steak	4.2	258	8.5	Peas, frozen	1.6	58	2.6
Pork chop	4.2	180	7.2	Bread,			
Cheese,				wholemeal	4.1*	108	1.8
cheddar	0.1	367	6.2	Potatoes	0.6	52	1.5

NB: All amounts are mg/100g.
*The niacin in wholemeal bread is unavailable to the body – hence niacin equivalent figure comes from tryptophan contribution only.

Reasons To Supplement

Alcoholics are commonly deficient in niacin and often need to be given a supplement of this vitamin – preferably along with other members of the B-complex.

Niacin (as nicotinic acid) has been used to very good effect in the lowering of blood fat levels. However, 'megadoses' (usually grammes per day) need to be used for this purpose and any such supplementation should therefore only be done under full medical supervision.

NB: Only nicotinic acid (*not* niacinamide) can lower blood fat levels.

High levels of niacin have been advocated in certain schizophrenic conditions and although the information on this subject is conflicting, there are reported cases of quite remarkable recoveries using niacin.

Osteoarthritis and other painful joint conditions may also respond to niacin treatment (as niacinamide).

How Safe?

Very high doses of nicotinic acid (3–6g per day) may cause changes in liver structure, with the timed-release form of the vitamin seeming more likely to be implicated in this respect. As a precaution, the Health Food Manufacturers' Association has recommended that timed-release nicotinic acid supplements should be removed from the market, and that non-timed-release supplements of nicotinic acid be limited to dosages of 100mg per day.

Niacinamide supplements are considered safe at levels up to 2,000mg per day.

Interactions With Other Substances

At levels above 20mg, nicotinic acid (*not* niacinamide) may cause dilation of blood vessels in the skin with resultant skin flushing. This effect usually wears off after days of repeated administration and occurs to a much lesser degree if the nicotinic acid is taken with food.

Supplements of nicotinic acid should not be taken by people suffering from the following conditions:

- Gout.
- Diabetes.
- Stomach ulcers.
- Liver disease.

PANTOTHENIC ACID

The name pantothenic acid comes from the word *panthos* meaning 'everywhere'. As its Greek name implies, it is widely available in all plant and animal tissue. It was first isolated from rice husks in 1939 and was first recognized as a factor required to prevent chickens from developing a form of dermatitis. Pantothenic acid is a water-soluble vitamin and a member of the B-complex.

The vitamin is normally presented in supplement form as calcium pantothenate (vitamin B5). Calcium pantothenate and pantothenic acid can be considered synonymous terms from the point of view of vitamin activity.

Pantothenic acid is destroyed by heat, acid (e.g. vinegar) or alkali (e.g. bicarbonate). The vitamin is also lost through leaching into cooking water.

What Does It Do?

Pantothenic acid is a part of the coenzyme A molecule that plays such an important part in the process of releasing energy from foods (fat, carbohydrates, and protein). Pantothenic acid is also of great importance in the function of the adrenal gland, and in the formation of antibodies.

Signs of Deficiency

A major deficiency of pantothenic acid does not cause a well defined deficiency disease. However, an affliction known as 'burning feet syndrome' noted amongst prisoners of war and malnourished subjects in the Far East is known to respond to administration of pantothenic acid.

Human subjects who have voluntarily deprived themselves of pantothenic acid describe developing symptoms of fatigue, headache, dizziness, muscle weakness and gastro-intestinal disturbance.

How Much?

The COMA 1991 report *Dietary Reference Values for Food Energy and Nutrients for the United Kingdom* does not give any specific recommendations for intake of pantothenic acid. This is because no acceptable biochemical method has yet been developed to accurately measure pantothenic acid status in humans.

However, an adequate intake of pantothenic acid by adults is thought to be 3–7mg daily. An adequate content of pantothenic acid in infant formulae is considered to be 2mg/litre (equivalent to 1.7mg per day or 3mg/1000kcal).

Food Sources

Food	Pantothenic Acid (mg/100g)	Food	Pantothenic Acid (mg/100g)
Brewer's yeast	9.5	Wheat bran	2.4
Pig's liver	6.5	Wheatgerm	2.2
Yeast extract	3.8	Eggs	1.8
Nuts	2.7	Poultry	1.2

Reasons To Supplement

Applied topically, good results have been claimed for pantothenic acid in the healing of bed sores and varicose ulcers. Given by injection, pantothenic acid has also shown promise in the prevention and treatment of paralytic ileus (intestinal obstruction resulting from decreased peristaltic activity in the bowel).

Due to its known role in the health of the adrenal gland and in the production of corticosteroid hormones, pantothenic acid is often advocated as a nutritional supplement to help the body cope with stress. It also may help to reduce allergic reactions in the respiratory and digestive systems.

Pantothenic acid may also be taken by sufferers from rheumatoid arthritis. It has been shown that this group of people are much more likely to have low levels of pantothenic acid in their blood. Moreover, studies assessing the effect of a pantothenic acid supplement in rheumatoid arthritis have yielded encouraging results.

How Safe?

No toxic signs were noted in young men given 10g of calcium pantothenate daily for six weeks, but such doses may cause diarrhoea and gastro-intestinal disturbances.

Interactions With Other Substances

It is usually recognized that B vitamins are best taken together for most general purposes. However, there is no detriment in taking pantothenic acid singly for a specific reason.

PYRIDOXINE

Pyridoxine or vitamin B6 is a well-known member of the water-soluble B group. Besides pyridoxine, two other variations on B6 exist – namely pyridoxal and pyridoxamine. All three forms exist routinely in animal and plant foods and have equal vitamin B6 activity.

Vitamin B6 is fairly resistant to heat but may leach out into water, and is also lost by exposure to alkalis or ultra-violet light.

What Does It Do?

Vitamin B6 is rapidly converted in the body to the coenzymes pryridoxal phosphate and pyridoxamine phosphate. These coenzymes play an essential role in protein metabolism, and also function in energy production, fat metabolism, central nervous system activity and haemoglobin production.

How Much?

The RNI Values (COMA 1991) for Vitamin B6 *

Age	(mg/day)	Age	(mg/day)
0–6 months	0.2	11–14 years (males)	1.2
7–9 months	0.3	11+ years (female)	1.0
10–12 months	0.4	15–18 years (males)	1.5
1–3 years	0.7	19+ years (males)	1.4
4–6 years	0.9		
7–10 years	1.0		

* Based on a protein intake that provides 14.7% of the estimated average energy intake.

Individuals with particularly high intakes of protein will need correspondingly more vitamin B6 in the diet.

Signs of Deficiency

The administration of a vitamin B6 antagonist to the diet of human volunteers produced symptoms of seborrhoea (oily skin with crusts and scales) around the eyes, nose and mouth. There was also a lowering of white blood cell count and a loss of ability to convert tryptophan to nicotinic acid. A type of anaemia was also noted.

Reasons To Supplement

There are various categories of people that tend to be deficient in vitamin B6 and could therefore benefit from a supplement of this vitamin. These include:

- Women on the contraceptive pill/hormone replacement therapy. (Many women on the contraceptive pill find vitamin B6 is a useful supplement to take as it can help alleviate the depression sometimes associated with taking this medication.)
- Pregnant women.
- Alcoholics.
- Smokers.

Supplemental vitamin B6 can also be useful in the treatment of PMT, and is used by many women for this purpose. Studies in this area have conflicting results, but 50–200mg daily does seem to be generally of benefit.

Vitamin B6 has been used for the prevention and treatment of nausea and vomiting due to irradiation, drug therapy, anaesthesia and in travel sickness, but a good response is not always seen.

Food Sources

The main sources of vitamin B6 in the diet are potatoes and other vegetables, milk and meat.

Food	Vitamin B6 (mg/100g)	Food	Vitamin B6 (mg/100g)
Wheatgerm	0.95	Potatoes	0.25
Bananas	0.51	Bread, wholemeal	0.12
Turkey	0.44	Baked beans	0.12
Chicken	0.29	Peas, frozen	0.10
Fish, white	0.29	Bread, white	0.07
Beef, stewing steak	0.27	Oranges	0.06
Brussels sprouts	0.28	Milk	0.06

How Safe?

2–7g of vitamin B6 daily may bring about the development of sensory neuropathy (numbness and tingling of nerves in the extremities). Such symptoms have also been reported in women taking as little as 50mg daily, but these reports have since largely been discredited. All cases of peripheral neuropathy disappeared within six months on withdrawal of the vitamin.

The most well accepted reasonable and safe dosage of vitamin B6 on a daily basis is about 100mg.

Interactions With Other Substances

It is usually recognized that B vitamins are best taken together for most general purposes. However, there is no detriment in taking vitamin B6 singly for a specific reason.

Vitamin B6 is not compatible with the Parkinson's disease medication levadopa, nor with the anti-convulsant medicines phenytoin and phenobarbitone.

COBALAMIN

Vitamin B12 contains cobalt and it is hence known as cobalamin. It is another member of the water-soluble B-complex, and is sometimes known as 'anti-pernicious' factor after its ability to prevent the condition pernicious anaemia.

The absorption of vitamin B12 is dependent on the presence of a certain substance known as 'intrinsic factor' in the gastric juices.

Vitamin B12 is freely soluble and therefore lost into cooking water. It is sensitive to strong acid, alkali and light. Particular care has to be taken in the formulation of a multivitamin tablet containing vitamin B12 because it is particularly sensitive to attack by other nutrients.

What Does It Do?

Vitamin B12 is needed at a very basic level for the synthesis of DNA and hence for cell production – particularly red blood cells.

Vitamin B12 also functions in the metabolism of fatty acids, and in maintaining the myelin sheath around the nerves.

Signs of Deficiency

A deficiency of vitamin B12 leads inevitably to the condition pernicious anaemia. This is characterized by a fall in the number of red blood cells. Those still produced are irregular in size, but generally too big.

Unfortunately there is an unpleasant twist to vitamin B12 deficiency, in that symptoms of pernicious anaemia can be effectively masked if folic acid intake is adequate. This can allow vitamin B12 deficiency to progress silently, showing itself eventually in irreversible neurological damage.

How Much?

The RNI Values (COMA 1991) for Vitamin B12

Age	(mcg/day)	Age	(mcg/day)
0–6 months	0.3	7–10 years	1.0
7–12 months	0.4	11–14 years	1.2
1–3 years	0.5	15+ years	1.5
4–6 years	0.8	Lactation	2.0

Food Sources

Food	Vitamin B12 (mcg/100g)	Food	Vitamin B12 (mcg/100g)
Lamb's liver	54.0	Fortified breakfast cereal	1.7
Pig's liver	23.0	Eggs	1.7
Fish, white	2.0	Yeast extract	0.5
Beef, lamb, pork	2.0		

Reasons To Supplement

Any one of the following categories of people may be deficient in vitamin B12 and require a supplement of this vitamin:

- Those with a deficiency of intrinsic factor who therefore cannot absorb the vitamin.
- Those with bacterial or parasitic infections which interfere with the normal absorption of vitamin B12 from the gut.
- Those with specific defects in the intestinal cell wall which prevent the normal absorption of vitamin B12.
- Vegans. (Vitamin B12 does not normally occur in vegetables.)
- Alcoholics.

The first three above are medical conditions that need suitably drastic treatment. To treat or prevent pernicious anaemia in these patients, vitamin B12 is often injected intramuscularly in large amounts. Through this method, pernicious anaemia has changed from being a fatal to a treatable disease.

Vegans and vegetarians may do well to supplement orally with vitamin B12. This is a suitable precaution because of the absence of this vitamin from plant foods.

High levels of vitamin B12 have also been used therapeutically for reasons other than treating pernicious anaemia. Certain mental conditions (especially in the aged) have been seen to be improved with vitamin B12, but there is no hard evidence for this.

How Safe?

No toxic effects have been noted with vitamin B12 in man. Injections of as much as 3mg/day have been used to treat fatigue and various neurological disorders.

FOLIC ACID

Folic acid was originally found in yeast, where it was recognized to be an 'anti-anaemia' factor. Folic acid is a member of the B-complex and has the chemical name pteroyl glutamic acid.

Folic acid is unstable to heat, air, water and alkali, and careful cooking methods must be employed to ensure adequate amounts of this vitamin are retained.

Deficiency

Those who are most at risk from folic acid deficiency are as follows:

- The elderly (who tend to have poorer diets or impaired absorption).
- Those with intestinal malabsorption syndromes (particularly steatorrhoea, where the stools contain undigested fat).
- Pregnant women (the developing foetus makes considerable demands on the maternal folic acid stores).
- Alcoholics.

Rapidly generating tissues are affected by folic acid deficiency and so the intestinal mucosa may also suffer. In babies and young children, growth may be affected.

In pregnant women, a deficiency of folic acid can be particularly harmful because it is undeniably associated with birth defects, especially spina bifida.

It is also acknowledged that folic acid deficiency can cause mental deterioration.

What Does It Do?

Folic acid is needed for many physiological reactions. More specifically, folic acid is needed for the synthesis of DNA and therefore for cell division. It is also involved in the metabolism of amino acids methionine and glycine.

Reasons To Supplement

Supplements of folic acid are highly advised prior to conception as well as during pregnancy, as low folic acid intake is strongly associated with the birth defect, spina bifida.

Folic acid supplements must be used under medical supervision for the treatment of diagnosed megaloblastic anaemia, as folic acid can mask a vitamin B12 deficiency (see vitamin B12). Normally, folic acid is only prescribed after vitamin B12 has already failed to bring a response.

Alcoholics may benefit from a supplement of folic acid as they tend to have depleted levels of this vitamin.

How Much?

The RNI Values (COMA 1991) for Folic Acid

Age	(mcg/day)	Age	(mcg/day)
0–12 months	50	11+ years	200
1–3 years	70	Pregnancy	300
4–6 years	100	Lactation	260
7–10 years	150		

Food Sources

Food	Folic Acid (mcg/100g)	Food	Folic Acid (mcg/100g)
Brewer's yeast	2,400	Bread, wholemeal	39
Wheatgerm	310	Eggs	30
Wheat bran	260	Bread, white	27
Nuts	110	Fish, fatty	26
Pig's liver	110	Bananas	22
Leafy green vegetables	90	Potatoes	14
Pulses	80		

How Safe?

The overall danger risk from folic acid mega-dosing is deemed very slight.

Interactions With Other Substances

As previously mentioned, folic acid supplements taken by people with developing vitamin B12 deficiency may obscure a correct diagnosis and delay the appropriate treatment. Very high folic acid intakes may also result in disturbed zinc absorption.

BIOTIN

Biotin is the eighth and final true B vitamin which was first discovered as the factor that protected against the toxicity of raw egg whites. Subsequently, it was found that there existed a biotin-binding factor in egg white – the effect of which was overcome by adding biotin to the diet.

What Does It Do?

Like many of the other B vitamins, biotin is involved in the intermediary metabolism of carbohydrates, energy and fats. It is of central importance in lipogenesis (fat manufacture), gluconeogenesis (glycogen manufacture), and branched chain amino acid metabolism.

Signs of Deficiency

Specific biotin deficiency is rare in human adults except in those who have consumed large amounts of raw eggs. The symptoms then show themselves as fine scaly dermatitis and hair loss. More extreme experimental depletion of biotin leads to anorexia, nausea, depression and hallucinations. All these symptoms are reversible upon injection of biotin.

Biotin deficiency is more common in babies and leads to the skin conditions seborrhoeic dermatitis and desquamating erythroderma (Leiner's disease).

How Much?

Current knowledge about biotin is insufficient for definitive dietary recommendations to be made. However the COMA 1991 report *Dietary Reference Values for Food Energy and Nutrients for the United Kingdom* suggests that intakes between 10 and 200mcg are both safe and adequate.

At present the average intake of biotin by British men is 39mcg/day (range 15–70mcg) and the average intake of biotin by British women is 26mcg/day (range 10–58mcg).

Food Sources

Food	Biotin (mcg/100g)	Food	Biotin (mcg/100g)
Brewers yeast	80	Chicken	10
Pig's kidney	32	Lamb	6
Yeast extract	27	Bread, wholemeal	6
Pig's liver	27	Fish, fatty	5
Wheat bran	14	Milk	2
Eggs, cooked (each)	12	Cheese	2
Wheatgerm	12		

Reasons To Supplement

Biotin brings rapid relief of seborrhoeic dermatitis and Leiner's disease in children suffering from these diseases.

Biotin supplements are sometimes recommended to candida albicans sufferers, because it is thought that biotin may prevent candida from changing into its invasive fungal form.

How Safe?

Biotin has been administered to infants in dosages of up to 40mg without side effects and so is regarded as a perfectly safe vitamin even at extremely high levels.

Interactions With Other Substances

It is usually recognized that B vitamins are best taken together for most general purposes. However there is no detriment in taking biotin singly if desired.

CHOLINE AND INOSITOL

The substances choline and inositol are sometimes loosely classified as 'B-complex factors' but they are not in fact true vitamins because they can be made in the body.

What Does It Do?

Choline and inositol are both components of various phospholipids – structural components within cell walls. They are also both strong lipotrophic factors, helping to prevent conditions such as fat infiltration of the liver.

Choline stimulates the production of lecithin, and is also part of the neurotransmitter acetylcholine which is vital to nerve impulse transmission.

Inositol functions to mediate the cells' response to certain stimuli including nerve impulses. It is also found very richly in male reproductive organs, particularly semen.

Food Sources

Food	Choline (mg/100g)	Inositol (mg/100g)	Food	Choline (mg/100g)	Inositol (mg/100g)
Liver, desiccated	2,170	1,100	Nuts	220	180
Heart, beef	1,720	1,600	Pulses	120	160
Liver	650	340	Citrus fruits	85	210
Beef steak	600	260	Bread, wholemeal	80	100
Brewer's yeast	300	50	Bananas	44	120

Reasons To Supplement

Choline and inositol may be used in supplement form to 'scour' deposited or circulating lipids from the body. Particularly, people with fatty liver or atherosclerotic plaques may benefit from choline and inositol.

NB: Choline and inositol are not designed to be slimming aids.

How Safe?

No toxic dose has ever been reported with inositol. Choline is also very safe, but at very high levels may cause a fishy smell through the skin and on the breath. There are also a few reports of choline exacerbating depression at several grammes a day.

Interactions With Other Substances

There are no reported drug interactions or contra-indications for choline or inositol.

PABA (PARA-AMINOBENZOIC ACID)

PABA is often thought of as a member of the B-complex but is not a true vitamin for man. PABA is part of the structure of folic acid.

What Does It Do?

The functions of PABA in humans are as yet not fully understood, but it appears to be involved in the metabolism of amino acids and red blood cells.

Food Sources

Not many figures are produced on the amount of PABA in food. However, liver, eggs, wheatgerm and molasses are known to be good sources.

Reasons To Supplement

Apart from its inclusion at low levels in multivitamin supplements, the major accepted use of PABA is as a remedy for vitiligo (a condition characterized by de-pigmentation of the skin).

PABA has been used in scleroderma (thickening of the skin) and in lupus erythematosus – another severe skin disorder. However, the dosages used in clinical trials for these conditions were extremely high and should not be self-administered.

PABA is also used topically applied as a sunscreen agent, but there is no evidence to say that it works internally for this purpose.

How Safe?

PABA appears quite safe at most dosage levels, but recent studies show 8g or more daily may cause malaise, fever and liver complaints.

Interactions With Other Substances

It is usually recognized that PABA is best taken together with the B-complex for most purposes. However there is no detriment in taking PABA singly for short periods if desired.

VITAMIN C (ASCORBIC ACID)

Vitamin C was first isolated in 1928 by Dr Szent Gyorgi, who was awarded a Nobel Prize for his discovery. James Lind confirmed the link between scurvy and vitamin C in 1768. English sailors were named 'limeys' because of the limes they carried aboard. They used lime juice as a supplement to prevent scurvy.

Some nine million people take vitamin C supplements in the UK, making it the most widely used supplement in the country.

Vitamin C is an unstable water-soluble vitamin which is sensitive to heat, air, water (by leaching), and alkali (e.g. bicarbonate of soda). Certain metals, such as copper, also speed the oxidative destruction of vitamin C.

What Does It Do?

Vitamin C has very many functions in the body – some still not completely understood. Below are listed some of the processes in which it is involved:

- Formation of collagen – the body's intercellular 'cement'.

- Growth, tissue repair and wound healing.
- Formation of antibodies and stimulation of the white blood cells.
- Formation of corticosteroid hormones in the adrenal glands.
- Oxidation of certain amino acids including tyrosine.
- Absorption of iron and its necessary accumulation in the bone marrow, spleen and liver.
- Metabolism of folic acid.

Vitamin C carries out most of its functions through acting as a powerful antioxidant. This also means that vitamin C is a very effective neutralizer of free radicals – destructive and highly reactive molecules that are thought to be the basis of many serious diseases including cancer and heart disease.

Signs of Deficiency

The classic vitamin C deficiency disease is scurvy, early symptoms of which are usually bleeding of the gums and loosening of the teeth, together with lassitude, weakness, irritability and muscle ache.

A prolonged marginal deficiency of vitamin C may not lead to clinical symptoms, but may predispose towards cancer and heart disease.

How Much?

It is well known that smoking severely depletes vitamin C – and the American Recommended Dietary Allowances take account of this by suggesting an intake of 100mg per day for smokers (their standard Daily Allowance is 60mg for adults).

The RNI Values (COMA 1991) for Vitamin C

Age	(mg/day)	Age	(mg/day)
0–12 months	25	15+ years	40
1–10 years	30	Pregnancy	50
11–14 years	35	Lactation	70

Food Sources

Food	Vitamin C (mg/100g)	Food	Vitamin C (mg/100g)
Blackcurrants	200	Tomatoes	20
Pepper, green	100	Potatoes	
Brussels sprouts	90	new	16
Mango	80	Oct–Dec	19
Cauliflower	60	Jan–Feb	9
Cabbage	55	Mar–May	8
Oranges	50	Lettuce	15
Grapefruit	40	Bananas	10
Sweet potatoes	25		

The main sources of vitamin C in the diet are potatoes, fruit juice, citrus fruit and green vegetables. The Vitamin C content of foods varies very widely depending upon season, variety and freshness.

Reasons To Supplement

Vitamin C is obviously a quick effective treatment for scurvy, but fortunately this disease is not often seen these days in Western countries, except perhaps in old people with a very poor intake of fresh fruit and vegetables.

There are many more situations in which vitamin C supplementation can have a therapeutic effect, some of which are detailed below. Around 1g/day would normally be recommended, although more may be taken.

Infection Controlled studies have shown that Vitamin C levels become depleted during the course of an infection. There is also evidence that large doses can help be preventative against the common cold.

Surgery and Fracture Vitamin C helps in wound healing after invasive surgery and is also vital for proper healing of fractures.

Dental and Oral Conditions Vitamin C given before and after dental extraction has been shown to result in rapid healing of gums.

Anaemia and Haemorrhagic Disorders   The use of vitamin C as an adjunct to anaemia treatment is well accepted because of the vitamin's important connection with iron metabolism. In haemorrhagic disorder, vitamin C may help to strengthen fragile capillaries, especially in conjunction with bioflavonoids (substances which are often found naturally occurring alongside vitamin C).

Osteoarthritis   Vitamin C (preferably in its buffered form) may be of benefit to sufferers from osteoarthritis, presumably through its role in collagen production. It seems to relieve the pain and stiffness in some people.

Allergies   Allergic conditions may be helped through vitamin C supplementation, presumably through an anti-histamine effect.

Stomach and Duodenal Ulcers   Vitamin C is very important to the healing of ulcers, but the 'buffered' (non-acidic) form should be used.

Safety

Vitamin C is on the whole extremely safe, with no toxic effects even at dosages of several grammes per day. Transient diarrhoea is the usual side effect that is noted when one takes more than the body can tolerate.

Interactions With Other Substances
It is not advisable for people with kidney stones to take high level Vitamin C (above approximately 1g per day).

Taking very high dosages of vitamin C – 5000mg a day and up – and then suddenly stopping the supplementation has been thought to possibly cause 'rebound scurvy'. However a recent review has shown there is no real basis for this belief. Nevertheless it is perhaps advisable to come off high level vitamin C slowly.

Vitamin C may possibly dilute the effect of tricyclic anti-depressants (e.g. amitriptyline, imipramine).

Various drugs may increase the need for Vitamin C, including cortisones, aspirin and birth control pills.

127

VITAMIN D (CALCIFEROL)

There are two main versions of this important fat-soluble vitamin – namely vitamin D2 and vitamin D3. Vitamin D3 (cholecalciferol) is made by the action of sunlight on cholesterol deposits in the skin, and is also found in animal liver oils. Vitamin D2 (ergocalciferol) is a vegetarian form of the vitamin formed from the action of ultra violet light on the precursor ergosterol. This is the only vitamin that is required in greater quantities by children than adults.

Vitamin D is measured in mcg and i.u. with the conversion factor being: 1i.u. = 40mcg.

Vitamin D is stable to normal cooking procedures.

What Does It Do?

Vitamin D is converted in the body to an important calcium-controlling hormone and all its functions are related to this hormone's effects.

The principle action of vitamin D hormone is to increase the absorption of calcium and phosphorus from the intestine and to promote the uptake of these minerals by bone. However, to maintain the body's physiological ratio of calcium to phosphorus vitamin D hormone also increases the excretion of phosphorus – but not calcium – from the kidneys.

Signs of Deficiency

Deficiency of vitamin D during childhood leads to the development of rickets. Rickets may show itself as early as two months of age, when 'craniotabes' (areas of softening on the skull) are noted. Production of the first teeth may be delayed and the posture affected. Rickets also produces enlargement at the ends of long bones, resulting in characteristic bowing of the legs when the child starts to walk.

In adults, deficiency of vitamin D leads to osteomalacia. This disease is essentially the same as rickets, but the symptoms are slightly different because the bones are not still developing. In osteomalacia, there is thinning and weakening of the bone and spontaneous fractures may occur.

These days, rickets and osteomalacia are fortunately not very

common in developed countries, especially as multivitamin supplements suitable for babies and children are so widely advocated
and available.

How Much?

The RNI Values (COMA 1991) for Vitamin D

Age	(mcg/day)	(i.u./day)	Age	(mcg/day)	(i.u./day)
0–6 months	8.5	340	Pregnancy	10	400
7 months–3 years	7	280	Lactation	10	400
65+ years	10	400			

It was decided by the COMA panel that in the 3-to-65-year age
group, vitamin D formed from skin exposure to the sun was usually
sufficient to satisfy needs, and that an extra dietary supply was
therefore generally unnecessary.

Food Sources

Food	Vitamin D (mcg/100g)	(i.u./100g)	Food	Vitamin D (mcg/100g)	(i.u./100g)
Cod liver oil	212.5	8,500	Butter	0.8	32
Herring and kipper	22.4	896	Liver	0.8	32
Salmon, canned	12.5	500	Cheese, cheddar	0.3	12
Milk, evaporated	4.0	160	Milk, whole	0.03	1.2
Eggs	1.6	64	Milk, skimmed	0	0

Reasons To Supplement

There are certain categories of people who are theoretically much
more likely to be at risk of vitamin D deficiency and who may
therefore need to supplement with this nutrient. These include:

- Vegetarians and especially vegans (vitamin D is found mostly
  in animal and dairy products).

- Asian women and children who may not eat many vitamin D containing foods and who choose to cover up their skin.
- Lactating women whose breastmilk can be low in Vitamin D especially during the winter.
- The housebound elderly with a tendency to eat poorly.

How Safe?

There are some reports of hypercalcaemia occurring in infants at a level of 50mcg (2,000i.u) vitamin D a day. In adults, symptoms of vitamin D toxicity have been reported at daily intakes of 625mcg (25,000i.u.).

However, there is also some early evidence that vitamin D at lower levels may have adverse effects unrelated to hypercalcaemia. As a guideline, a maximum of 1,000i.u. vitamin D should be taken daily unless under medical advice.

Interactions With Other Substances

Vitamin D and vitamin A are found together in many food sources, although they are not actually dependent upon one another for their absorption or utilization.

When digitoxin and certain other cardiac glycoside heart drugs are taken in combination with vitamin D, there is a slight risk of abnormal heart rhythm.

VITAMIN E (TOCOPHEROL)

Fat soluble vitamin E was originally discovered to be a fertility factor for animals, but our knowledge about its functions have since progressed in leaps and bounds. Much research has gone into vitamin E's potential therapeutic and preventative uses. There are several food substances called tocopherols which are collectively known as vitamin E. The word 'tocopherol' comes from two Greek words – *tokos* meaning birth and *phero* meaning 'to bear', and it is also known as a fertility vitamin.

Vitamin E actually consists of four substances: alpha, beta, delta and gamma tocopherol. There are natural and synthetic forms of all the tocopherols. The naturally occurring form of vitamin E is the 'D' form, as in D-alpha tocopherol. The synthetic form is the 'DL' form as in DL-alpha tocopherol. The 'D' form is a much more absorbable form of Vitamin E.

Vitamin E supplements may contain alpha alone, but can also contain mixed tocopherols. Mixed tocopherol supplements are the ideal, since they represent the way vitamin E exists naturally in food.

Commercial food processing reduces the vitamin E content of foods as do freezing and deep frying. Solvent extraction of vegetable oils also destroys vitamin E.

What Does It Do?

Vitamin E has a very powerful antioxidant effect in the body – protecting the lipids in cell walls particularly. Lipids are particularly susceptible to oxidation by free radicals (highly reactive by-products of metabolism also arising from environmental sources).

In its capacity as an antioxidant, vitamin E can act to reduce the oxygen requirement of muscles and thereby increase exercise capacity. It also helps healing and is protective against atherosclerosis and thrombosis.

Vitamin E also has an important neurological role and prevents degeneration of the nerves and muscles.

Signs of Deficiency

Deficiency of vitamin E does not lead to any specific disease in the short term, but chronic insufficiency of vitamin E is thought to be a contributory factor in cancer and heart disease.

In children, fat malabsorption can lead to a deficiency of vitamin E characterized by abnormal red blood cell development.

How Much?

The requirement for vitamin E is determined to a large extent by the polyunsaturated fatty acid (PUFA) content of the diet. The COMA 1991 panel on *Dietary Reference Values* felt that PUFA intakes in Britain varied so widely that it was impossible to set RNIs. Also, people's individual requirements for vitamin E vary dramatically.

Nevertheless, although there is no general agreement on what factor should be used, 0.4mg vitamin E/g of dietary PUFA has been assessed to be adequate in American diets. Assuming PUFA intake provides 6% of dietary energy, this means the intake of vitamin E by 18–50-year-old males should be 7mg/day, and the intake of vitamin E by 18–50-year-old females should be 5mg/day.

Food Sources

Food	Vitamin E (mg/100g)	Food	Vitamin E (mg/100g)
Wheatgerm oil	178	Peanut butter	9
Safflower oil	97	Soybean oil	8
Sunflower seeds, raw	74	Butter	3
Sunflower oil	73	Asparagus	2.7
Almonds	37	Spinach	2.7
Mayonnaise	19	Broccoli	0.7
Wheatgerm	17	Bananas	0.3
Margarine, hard	16	Strawberries	0.3

Reasons To Supplement

Vitamin E supplements are advised in individuals who have fat malabsorption problems.

To date, these are some of the conditions that vitamin E supplements may help to prevent:

- Heart problems (atherosclerosis, angina, thrombosis, elevated cholesterol, and so on).
- Cancer. *
- Cataracts. *
- Circulatory disorders.
- Fibrocystic breast disease.
- Blood platelet aggregation (for instance, in susceptible women on the contraceptive pill).
- Parkinson's disease.

*It is strictly illegal to recommend any product whatsoever for the treatment of cancer and cataracts.

Vitamin E may also be used as a nutritional therapy in the following conditions:

- PMT (especially with evening primrose oil).
- Post-operative wound healing.
- Poor circulation, varicose veins etc.

How Safe?

Vitamin E is thought to be safe at levels up to 3,200mg per day. Levels over about 800i.u. vitamin E (D-alpha tocopherol) have occasionally been associated with such symptoms as fatigue, nausea, mild gastro-intestinal problems, palpitations and transient blood pressure increase. Such symptoms are reversible and to minimize any possibility of adverse effects, increasing up to this level may be done slowly.

Interactions With Other Substances

Vitamin E supplements should only be taken under medical supervision by people on anti-coagulant drugs. High levels of vitamin E are also best avoided by diabetics and those with hypothyroidisim.

Vitamin E activity is increased by selenium and vice versa.

CALCIUM

Calcium is the most abundant mineral in the human body, comprising over 1.5% of the total body weight. About 99% of the body's calcium is found in the bones, with the remaining 1% in the soft tissues. Calcium absorption is vitally dependent upon vitamin D, and consequently vitamin D and calcium deficiency symptoms are often synonymous.

Reasons To Supplement

Calcium may be taken by anyone who is worried that they may be at risk of calcium deficiency. This could include:

- Vegetarians and especially vegans.
- Young women with a history of osteoporosis in the family.

- Post-menopausal women.
- Pregnant and lactating women.
- Users of aluminium-containing antacids (indigestion pills or powders) which deplete calcium.

How Much?

The RNI Values (COMA 1991) for Calcium

Age	(mg/day)	Age	(mg/day)
0–12 months	525	11–18 years (males)	1,000
1–3 years	350	11–18 years (females)	800
4–6 years	450	19+ years	700
7–10 years	550	Lactation	1,250

Food Sources

Food	Calcium (mg/100g)	Food	Calcium (mg/100g)
Skimmed milk powder	1,230	Natural yoghurt	200
Cheese, cheddar	800	Milk, whole	103
Sardines	550	Peanuts, roasted	61
Tofu	506	Cabbage	57
Dried figs	280	Bread, wholemeal	54
Evaporated milk	260	Eggs	52
Watercress	220	Fish, white	22

MAGNESIUM

Quantitatively, magnesium ranks next to phosphorus and calcium in the body. Magnesium is intimately involved with calcium in metabolism.

More than 65% of the magnesium content of the body is found in the bone, where along with calcium and phosphorus it provides structure and strength.

The mineral plays a pivotal role in energy release, as it is a cofactor in energy-producing reactions. It is also needed in RNA synthesis and in DNA replication – i.e. in cell production. Additionally, magnesium is important in the functioning of nerves and muscles.

How Much?

The RNI Values (COMA 1991) for Magnesium

Age	(mg/day)	Age	(mg/day)
0–3 months	55	7–10 years	200
4–6 months	60	11–14 years	280
7–9 months	75	15–18 years	300
10–12 months	80	19+ years (males)	300
1–3 years	85	19+ years (females)	270
4–6 years	120	Lactation	320

Food Sources

Food	Magnesium (mg/100g)	Food	Magnesium (mg/100g)
Peanuts, roasted	180	Beef, stewing steak	18
Bread, wholemeal	76	Potatoes	17
Cheese, cheddar	25	Oranges	13
Food	Magnesium (mg/100g)	Food	Magnesium (mg/100g)
Fish, white	23	Eggs	12
Chicken	21		

Reasons to Supplement

Magnesium is often taken by women to ease PMT, especially stomach cramps and sugar cravings. The use of magnesium in this situation makes a lot of sense because tests have borne out that blood magnesium levels do drop before a period.

Other conditions in which magnesium has been found to be

helpful are involuntary muscle twitches (of the eyelid for example) and combined with calcium for muscle cramps. Again in relation to muscle function, it is also thought that magnesium has some protective effect on the heart, perhaps more particularly in the prevention of arrhythmias (irregular heart beats).

IRON

Iron is the second most abundant mineral in the earth's crust after aluminium. It is also a very important mineral in human physiology, but is in fact only a trace mineral in terms of concentration in the body. (The body contains approximately 4–5g).

The main function of iron in the diet is as an important constituent of the blood pigment haemoglobin. Haemoglobin is contained within red blood cells and is the carrier of vital oxygen around the body. Other than its function in red blood cells, iron is also found in myoglobin (the equivalent of haemoglobin found in muscle) and is additionally a participant in energy-producing reactions of the body.

How Much?

The RNI Values (COMA 1991) for Iron

Age	(mg/day)	Age	(mg/day)
0–3 months	1.7	7–10 years	8.7
4–6 months	4.3	11–18 years (males)	11.3
7–12 months	7.8	11–50 years (females)	14.8
1–3 years	6.9	19–50 years (males)	8.7
4–6 years	6.1	50+ years	8.7

Reasons To Supplement

Women of childbearing age are at the most risk of iron deficiency because of their monthly menstrual blood losses. The RNIs above do not take into account those women with high menstrual losses, who are advised to meet their extra needs with a supplement.

Other people who may need an iron supplement include vegetarians, pregnant women, adolescents, athletes and the elderly.

A multivitamin and mineral supplement containing iron in a suitable balance with other nutrients is to be recommended for children, but iron at higher levels should not be taken by children except under medical advice.

Food Sources

Age	Iron (mg/100g)	Age	Iron (mg/100g)
Curry powder	29.6	Eggs	2.0
Fortified breakfast cereal	16.7	Beef	1.9
Lamb's liver	7.5	Watercress	1.6
Pig's kidney	6.4	Bread, white	1.6
Apricots, dried	4.1	Cabbage	0.6
Bread, wholemeal	2.7	Red wine	0.5
Corned beef	2.4	Fish, white	0.5
Chocolate, plain	2.4	Potatoes	0.4

POTASSIUM

Potassium is an electrolyte mineral which means that it has a part in controlling the fluid level and acid/alkaline balance of the body and its billions of cells. Potassium is kept inside the cell and is counter-balanced by sodium which remains outside the cell.

Reasons To Supplement

Potassium may be deficient in people who take certain diuretic medications, and such individuals may need to take a potassium supplement. However, a doctor's advice should be sought first, as not all diuretics deplete potassium and some may indeed encourage its retention within the body.

Athletes or manual workers can also lose significant amounts of potassium through sweat and may benefit from a potassium supplement together with other minerals (such as calcium and magnesium).

Long-term use of certain antibiotics (especially penicillin) may deplete potassium and make a supplement advisable.

For people in general good health and for whom the above situations do not apply, supplementation with potassium is not normally advised except as part of a full spectrum multivitamin and mineral tablet.

How Much?

The RNI Values (COMA 1991) for Potassium

Age	(mg/day)	Age	(mg/day)
0–3 months	800	4–6 years	1,100
4–6 months	850	7–10 years	2,000
7–12 months	700	11–14 years	3,100
1–3 years	800	15+ years	3,500

Food Sources

Food	Potassium (mg/100g)	Sodium (mg/100g)	Food	Potassium (mg/100g)	Sodium (mg/100g)
Instant coffee	3,780	81	Bread, wholemeal	230	560
Potato crisps	1,190	550	Peas, frozen	190	3
Raisins	860	52	Streaky bacon	183	1245
Potatoes	360	8	Oranges	180	2
Pork	360	65	Milk, whole	140	50
Cauliflower	350	8	Eggs	136	140
Tomatoes	290	3	Cheese, cheddar	120	610
Chicken	290	75			

ZINC

The zinc content of the adult body is approximately 2–3g, and the mineral is found most highly concentrated in the muscles, liver, kidneys and eyes. In males, zinc is also present in large amounts in the prostate gland and sperm.

138

A component of over eighty enzymes, zinc functions in more enzymatic reactions than any other trace mineral.

The RNI Values (COMA 1991) for Zinc

Age	(mg/day)	Age	(mg/day)
0–6 months	4.0	15+ years (males)	9.5
7 months – 3 years	5.0	15+ years (females)	7.0
4–6 years	6.5	Lactation (0–4 months)	13.0
7–10 years	7.0	(4+ months)	9.5
11–14 years	9.0		

Food Sources

Food	Zinc (mg/100g)	Food	Zinc (mg/100g)
Cheese, cheddar	4.0	Bread, white	0.6
Beef, stewing steak	3.8	Milk	0.4
Bread, wholemeal	1.8	Fish, white	0.4
Eggs	1.5	Potatoes, old	0.3
Chicken	1.1		

Reasons To Supplement

Zinc and Acne   During puberty, there is an increased requirement for zinc due to increased hormone production. Zinc supplementation has been shown to be as effective as tetracycline in some acne sufferers, but it will often take up to twelve weeks of supplementation before a really good improvement is noted.

Zinc and Rheumatoid Arthritis   Zinc supplementation can be beneficial in the pain and swelling of arthritis. This may be because of an interlink between zinc and essential fatty acid metabolism.

Zinc and Pregnancy   The zinc status of pregnant women may be suspect because of the demands of the foetus. Zinc supplements may be necessary with a doctor's approval, along with iron and folic acid.

Zinc and Vegetarians   In vegetarian diets, zinc tends not to be so available because phytate found in fibrous plant foods binds it up and makes it unavailable to the body. Vegetarians may therefore be advised to supplement with zinc, either on its own or as part of a multi-formula.

IODINE

Iodine forms part of the hormones thyroxine and triiodothyronine which are necessary for the maintenance of metabolic rate, cellular metabolism and integrity of the connective tissue.

How Much?

The RNI Values (COMA) 1991 for Iodine

Age	(mcg/day)	Age	(mcg/day)
0–3 months (formula fed)	50	7–10 years	110
4–12 months	60	11–14 years	130
1–3 years	70	15+ years	140
4–6 years	100		

Food Sources

No accurate picture can be given of the iodine content of plant foods because this is so highly dependent upon the soil in which they are grown. However, as a rough guide, up to a maximum of 10mcg/100g in vegetables and grains would be expected. The same figure would apply to most meats.

Fish is a rich source of iodine with amounts (in mcg/100g): haddock, 659; whiting, 65–361; herring 21–27. Kelp is the very richest source of iodine, containing up to 5,000mg or more per 100g.

Reasons To Supplement

Iodine in the form of kelp may be taken to stimulate a slightly underactive thyroid gland that does not warrant medical treatment.

More usually, iodine is included in small amounts in multi-formulae that are suitable for use by all normal healthy people.

MANGANESE

Manganese is an important trace mineral whose functions include:

- The development and maintenance of healthy bones.
- Sex hormone synthesis.
- Nerve development and function.
- Activation of natural killer cells.

How Much?

The COMA 1991 report on *Dietary Reference Values for Food Energy and Nutrients for the United Kingdom* does not give any RNIs for manganese, but suggests that safe intakes lie above 1.4mg per day for adults. Total manganese intakes in Britain are estimated at 4.6mg per day.

Food Sources

Tea is estimated to supply half the amount of manganese in the British diet. Otherwise, wholegrains, nuts and avocados are rich sources, with other fruits and vegetables containing moderate amounts. The milling of grains removes 73% of manganese.

Food	Manganese (mg/100g)	Food	Manganese (mg/100g)
Bread, wholemeal	4.3	Tea (1 cup)	1.5
Wheatgerm	4.2	Coconut	1.3
Avocados	4.2	Pineapple	1.1
Chestnuts	3.7	Plums	1.0
Hazelnuts	3.5	Lettuce	0.7
Peas	2.0	Bananas	0.6
Almonds	1.9	Beetroot	0.6

MOLYBDENUM

Functions

Molybdenum is necessary for the functioning of the enzyme xanthine oxidase which is involved in iron metabolism and also in the production of uric acid (a waste product found in the blood and urine). Molybdenum is also needed for normal sexual functioning in the male.

How Much?

The 1991 COMA panel on *Dietary Reference Values* set no RNIs for molybdenum, but believed safe intakes were between 50 and 400mcg.

Food Sources

Food	Molybdenum (mcg/100g)	Food	Molybdenum (mcg/100g)
Canned beans	350	Eggs	50
Wheatgerm	200	Rice	47
Liver	200	Noodles	45
Lentils	120	Chicken	40
Sunflower seeds	103	Bread, wholemeal	26
Kidney	75	Potatoes	25
Green beans	66	Shellfish	20
Macaroni	51	Apricots	14

Reasons To Supplement

Except in proven molybdenum deficiency, there are no known therapeutic uses of supplemental molybdenum except perhaps to detoxify excess copper. Molybdenum may however be included in a general multivitamin and mineral supplement to ensure a sufficiency of this mineral.

SELENIUM

Selenium's name is derived from the moon goddess, Selene. This trace mineral was at first regarded as a poison, until the discovery that it was in fact needed to prevent degeneration of liver tissue. Selenium carries out its main functions as part of the enzyme glutathione peroxidase. Glutathione peroxidase is an antioxidant which protects intracellular structures against oxidative damage by free radicals.

Selenium is known to have a role in the following:

- Preservation of normal liver function.
- Protection against cancer.
- Maintenance of a healthy heart.
- Inhibition of harmful effects from heavy metals such as arsenic, cadmium, mercury and lead.

Selenium deficiency has traditionally occurred in areas where the soil is particularly low in this mineral. However, as modern lifestyles have allowed us to eat foods from very many different countries of origin, true selenium deficiency has become less of a problem.

How Much?

The RNI Values (COMA 1991) for Selenium

Age	(mcg/day)	Age	(mcg/day)
0–3 months	10	11–14 years	45
4–6 months	13	15–18 years (males)	70
7–12 months	10	15+ years (females)	60
1–3 years	15	19+ years (males)	75
4–6 years	20	Lactation	75
7–10 years	30		

Reasons To Supplement

The groups of people particularly found to be at risk of selenium deficiency are as follows:

- Young adults (especially students not eating a balanced diet).
- Vegetarians.

- The elderly.
- Pregnant and nursing mothers.
- Smokers.

Food Sources

Food	Selenium (approx. mcg/100g)	Food	Selenium (approx. mcg/100g
Organ meats	40	Wholegrains and cereals	12
Fish and shellfish	32	Dairy products	5
Meat	18	Fruit and vegetables	2

VANADIUM

More research needs to be done before a definitive role is established for vanadium in human nutrition. However, it appears to be needed for normal growth, fertility and lipid metabolism.

How Much?

Dietary requirement has not been well defined, but the amount lost in the urine on a daily basis is approximately 10mcg and so at least this much is needed from the diet each day.

Food Sources

Food	Vanadium (mcg/100g)	Food	Vanadium (mcg/100g)
Parsley	2,950	Sardines	46
Lobster	1,610	Cucumber	38
Radishes	790	Apples	33
Dill	460	Cauliflower	9
Lettuce	280	Tomatoes	4
Strawberries	70	Potatoes	1

CHROMIUM

Chromium appears to function biologically in an organic complex that potentiates the action of insulin. The name of this organic complex is 'glucose tolerance factor'.

Chromium depletion has been implicated in high blood cholesterol levels and in poor glucose tolerance.

How Much?

Chromium was not given an RNI value by the COMA 1991 panel on *Dietary Reference Values for Food Energy and Nutrients in the United Kingdom*. However, a safe and adequate level is believed to lie above 25mcg per day.

Food Sources

Food	Chromium (mg/100g)	Food	Chromium (mg/100g)
Egg yolk	183	Honey	29
Molasses	121	Potatoes, old	27
Brewer's yeast	117	Wheatgerm	23
Beef	57	Chicken leg	18
Cheese	56	Spaghetti	15
Grape juice	47	Spinach	10
Bread, wholemeal	42	Bananas	10
Wheat bran	38	Haddock	7
Raw sugar	35	Milk, skimmed	2

Reasons To Supplement

Therapy with chromium has been successful in people suffering from glucose tolerance problems (e.g. in those tending towards diabetes).

Chromium has also been shown to help lower total cholesterol levels and increase beneficial HDL cholesterol.

Finally, new research indicates that chromium may be able to increase lean muscle mass in athletes.

COPPER

Copper is in itself an oxidant, yet in the body it has an antioxidant function by being a participant in the enzyme superoxide dismutase (SOD). This enzyme protects the cells from the damage caused by free radicals and peroxides.

Copper is also part of the protein, ceruloplasmin, found in the blood plasma. Ceruloplasmin regulates the level of certain hormones in the blood and is also required for the formation of red blood cells.

Additionally, copper plays a part in energy production, melanin (skin pigment) formation, and fatty acid oxidation.

How Much?

The RNI Values (COMA 1991) for Copper

Age	(mg/day)	Age	(mg/day)
9–12 months	0.3	11–14 years	0.8
1–3 years	0.4	15–16 years	1.0
4–6 years	0.6	18+ years	1.2
7–10 years	0.7	Lactation	1.5

Food Sources

Food	Copper (mg/100g)	Food	Copper (mg/100g)
Oysters	7.6	Hazelnuts	1.4
Whelks	7.2	Shrimps	0.8
Lamb's liver	6.0	Cod	0.6
Crab	4.8	Bread, wholemeal	0.25
Brewer's yeast	3.3	Peas	0.2
Olives	1.6		

Reasons To Supplement

A copper supplement may be necessary when zinc is being taken, as the latter depletes copper. Copper is also necessary in Menke's syndrome (a rare genetic disease characterized by the inability to absorb copper). However in the case of this condition, copper injections are often prescribed.

Copper may be useful in combating inflammatory diseases such as rheumatoid arthritis and osteoarthritis. Copper bangles are often worn by sufferers for this reason.

In healthy individuals, copper is normally only necessary at low levels in balance with other nutrients.

BORON

Boron is a trace mineral that has only recently been recognized as having relevance in human nutrition. Bones contain the highest concentrations of boron and the parathyroid and thyroid glands also accumulate this mineral.

The exact function of boron in human nutrition is yet to be fully understood. However, the mineral is thought to play a part in maintaining bone density.

How Much?

The daily requirement of boron has yet to be defined, as it is yet to be proven that this mineral is essential for life.

Reasons To Supplement

Based on the data available so far, it appears that boron has a remarkable effect on the prevention of bone loss and demineralization. In a study conducted at the USA Department of Agriculture, 3mg of boron given to menopausal women was found to depress the loss of calcium and magnesium in the urine and double levels of an oestrogen metabolite which is known to be a reliable agent for preventing calcium loss from bone.

The Australian researcher Newnham has also reported abatement of rheumatoid arthritis symptoms and speedier healing of broken bones with boron supplementation.

Food Sources

Vegetables are by far the richest source of boron. Dairy products, fish and meat are the next best sources (in that order). The boron content of most diets is 1.5–3 mg/day.

Food	Boron (mg/100g)	Food	Boron (mg/100g)
Soya Beans	2.8	Peanuts	1.8
Prunes	2.7	Hazelnuts	1.6
Raisins	2.5	Dates	0.92
Almonds	2.3	Wine	up to 0.85
Rosehips	1.9		

Further Reading

The Vitamin Bible, Dr Earl Mindell, Arlington Books, 1991.
Vitamins and your Health, Ann Gildroy, Unwin, 1982.
Viruses, Allergies and the Immune System, Jan de Vries, Mainstream, 1990.
Food Facts, Ebury Press, 1990.
Vitamin Vitality, Patrick Holford, Collins, 1985.
Complete Nutrition, Dr Michael Sharon, Prion, 1989.
Beta Carotene, Caroline Wheater, Thorsons, 1991.
The Premenstrual Syndrome, Dr Caroline Shreeve, Thorsons, 1983.

Further Information

Useful Addresses

Nutrition Society
10 Cambridge Court
210 Shepherd's Bush Road
London W6 7NJ

McCarrison Society
24 Paddington Street
London W1 4DR

Community Health Foundation
188 Old Street
London EC1V 9PB

The Nutrition Association
36 Wycombe Road
Marlow
Bucks SL7 3HX

National Association of Health Stores
Bastow House
Queens Road
Nottingham NG2 3AS

Nutritional Science Research Institute
Mulberry Tree Road
Brookthorpe
Gloucester GL4 0UU

Courses

Centre for Nutritional Studies
The Garden House
Rutford Abbey
Newark
Notts

College of Dietary Therapy
Hillsborough House
Ashley
Tiverton
Devon EX16 5 PA

Foundation for Applied Nutrition
133 Gately Road
Gately
Cheadle
Cheshire SK8 4PD

Institute of Optimum Nutrition
5 Jerdan Place
London SW6 1BE

International Academy of Nutrition
P.O. Box 8
Liphook
Hants SU30 7JD

International Institute of Vitamin &
    Mineral Therapists
3 Ryde Mews
Binstead Road
Ryde
Isle of Wight

Index